Clyde V. Kiser

# THE MILBANK MEMORIAL FUND:
## *Its Leaders and Its Work 1905-1974*

### *Errata*

| | |
|---|---|
| p. 25, l. 21 | "wich" should be "with" |
| p. 41, l. 3 | "his tory" should be "history" |
| p. 57, l. 7 | "hte" should be "the" |
| p. 87, l. 30 | "Boudeau" should be "Boudreau" |
| p. 98, l. 20 | "alloted" should be "allotted" |
| p. 99, l. 7 | "196" should be "1968" |
| p. 100, l. 18 | "Millbank" should be "Milbank" |
| p. 135, right-hand column, l. 14 | "give" should be "gave" |
| p. 157 | George Baehr, M.D., Number of Years on Board "2.7" should be "27" |
| p. 159 | Thomas J. Parran, Jr., M.D. Dates of Appointment/From "11/25/20" should be "11/25/30" Length of Appointment "1" should be "31" |
| p. 165 | "Margaret W. Bernard" should be "Margaret W. Barnard" |

*The*
# Milbank Memorial Fund

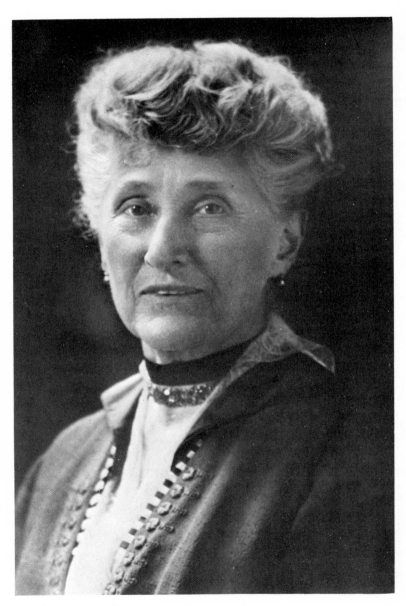

ELIZABETH MILBANK ANDERSON

# The
# Milbank Memorial Fund
## Its Leaders and Its Work
## 1905–1974

CLYDE V. KISER

Milbank Memorial Fund
New York
1975

Published for the Milbank Memorial Fund by
PRODIST
a division of
Neale Watson Academic Publications, Inc.
156 Fifth Avenue
New York 10010
© 1975 Milbank Memorial Fund
Designed and manufactured in U.S.A.


*Library of Congress Cataloging in Publication Data*

Kiser, Clyde Vernon, 1904–
   The Milbank Memorial Fund : its leaders and its work :
1905–1974.

   Includes index.
   1.   Milbank Memorial Fund.
HV97.M6K57            361.7′0973            74-20827
ISBN 0-88202-058-7

## CONTENTS

# Foreword

THE MILBANK MEMORIAL FUND is one of the oldest foundations in the United States. Founded in 1905 by Mrs. Elizabeth Milbank Anderson as the Memorial Fund Association, it was renamed the Milbank Memorial Fund and enlarged through additional sums bequeathed by Mrs. Anderson, after her death in 1921.

In a real sense, this is the history of Mrs. Anderson, a woman who was "involved in mankind" throughout her life. The Fund was her legacy to society, conceived and created to promote the public good. This history has another important purpose, to give an accounting of the stewardship of this legacy through almost seven decades. Perhaps the diary of a foundation as old as the Milbank Memorial Fund will provide additional meaning and substance to the historic as well as the current importance of foundations, expressing ancient cultures brought to this country by our forefathers, including initiative, creative diversity and pluralism, values as important today as they were in 1905.

From the beginning, the Fund's chief focus of activity has been —broadly interpreted—the area of public health. However, each of the five successive executive directors has been interested in somewhat different aspects of this field.

Although several brief histories of the Fund have been written, the last published (apart from brief summaries presented at Annual Conferences) covered only the period 1905–1940.

The author of the present account, Clyde V. Kiser, worked with the Milbank Memorial Fund for nearly 40 years, from 1931 to 1970. Beginning his career at the Fund in 1931 as a Research Fellow, he witnessed and participated in the Fund's pioneering efforts to demonstrate the relevance of population and family planning to public health. He is the only person who has served under all five executive directors of the Fund.

Dr. Kiser has chosen to organize his materials chronologically and to use the successive periods of directorship as chapter headings. Having worked with the Division of Research, he has emphasized the Fund's own research projects rather than its grants. It is hoped that the volume will be of interest to students of public health and demography as well as to the increasing number of people involved in the work of foundations.

L. E. Burney
President

# Preface

FREQUENTLY, when a man retires, his friends tell him he can now do what he wants to do. This book is a result of that new freedom.

Upon my retirement from the Milbank Memorial Fund, on 1 January 1971, I was given the opportunity to perform two pleasant tasks. The first was to organize a conference on the topic, "Forty Years of Research in Human Fertility: Retrospect and Prospect," which was to serve three major purposes: to honor my retirement, to memorialize the work of the Milbank Memorial Fund, and to attempt an objective evaluation of the research in population of the past forty years.

The other pleasant task was to write this history of the Milbank Memorial Fund. I hasten to add, however, that the word "pleasant" in this context must not be equated with such words as "easy," "recreational," or "child's play." Whether or not the final product appears to reflect the fact, much hard work, many difficult decisions, and many frustrations went into the writing of this book.

The task greatly increased my respect for historians. Whether they are concerned with the development of civilizations, cultures, governments, theories, political parties, or individuals, historians are frequently obliged to evaluate and choose between conflicting evidence.

One who undertakes to write a history of any foundation must decide upon a primary focus. He might concentrate upon the grants, the executive directors, the founder and the members of the Board, or an evaluation of the work of the foundation, or he might examine the foundation as an agent of social change, as an educational enterprise, or as a catalyst to encourage governmental agencies to undertake research or action in a particular field.

This present effort is not based exclusively on any one of these approaches—perhaps, to some extent, it uses all of them. As the chapter titles indicate, however, the fundamental approach is chronological, an effort to review the work of the Fund under its successive leaders. It begins with the forebears of the founder, Mrs. Elizabeth Milbank Anderson, and describes certain of her private philanthropies before the foundation was organized.

Chapter 2 concerns the Memorial Fund Association from the date of its organization in 1905 until 1921, when Mrs. Anderson died and the Association was renamed Milbank Memorial Fund.

Chapter 3 is devoted to the work of the Milbank Memorial Fund from 1922 to 1936, first under the direction of John A. Kingsbury and then of Edgar Sydenstricker. It depicts the origin, operation, and results of the New York Health Demonstrations. It also chronicles the founding of the Technical Board, the Advisory Council, the *Milbank Memorial Fund Quarterly*, the Annual Conferences, the Division of Research, and the Fund's pioneering entrance into research in several fields, including the sensitive areas of population, family planning, and medical care. Although Edgar Sydenstricker lived to serve as Scientific Director for only one year after Kingsbury's resignation in 1935, he had come to the Fund in 1926, and it was he who guided the early formative work of the Division of Research.

Chapter 4 presents a fairly detailed account of the work of the Fund during its twenty-five years (1937–1962) under the direction of Frank G. Boudreau. Here are described the development of the Fund's work in nutrition, housing, and mental health, the three fields which Dr. Boudreau introduced to the Fund, and the continuation of previous interests in various aspects of public health and population. In addition, this chapter tells of Dr. Boudreau's interest in international problems and of his role in the creation and development of the World Health Organization and the Food and Agriculture Organization of the United Nations.

Chapter 5 portrays the Fund's change of direction, from emphasis on research to one on medical education and preventive medicine, during the seven years (1962–1969) of the directorship of Dr. Alexander Robertson. Architect of the Fund's Milbank Faculty Fellowship Program, Dr. Robertson strove to use this project as a vehicle for improving medical education in the Americas, for promoting the ideas and ideals of social and preventive medicine, for developing medical leadership, and for encouraging the introduction of social science—including demography—into training for the health professions.

Briefly depicted in chapter 6 is the interregnum of 1969–1970, when a Technical Committee, composed of John S. Baugh, Per G. Stensland, and myself endeavored to "mind the store" until the appointment and inauguration of the next Executive Director.

Chapter 7 deals with the Fund's program of studies in the utilization of health services, under the direction of its current President, L. E. Burney. Plans for a three-year study of schools of public health are described in some detail, as are the phasing out of several traditional areas of interest to permit the orderly development of the new interests.

In chapter 8 may be found an overview of the Fund's sixty-nine years of existence, shown in terms of its changing structure, methods, and fields of interest. I have here taken the opportunity for a brief discussion of what seem to be possible sources of weakness and of strength in considering a foundation as an agency for change.

The Appendices present excerpts from documents, newspapers, and letters, together with lists of the names of past and present members of the Board of Directors, Technical Board, and professional and technical staff of the Fund that may be of historical interest.

I wish to thank, first of all, Dr. L. E. Burney for suggesting that this task be undertaken, for making available the necessary documents, and for providing facilities for accomplishing much of the work. John S. Baugh and other members of the staff have generously afforded their full cooperation. I am grateful to Dr. Ernest M. Gruenberg for his help in strengthening chapter 4 and to Dr. Bertram Brown, Dr. Morton Kramer, and Philip Hallen for their appraisals of the significance of the Fund's work in mental health. In particular, I wish to thank Miss Betty A. Vorwald and Miss Mary P. Mele for their arduous labor in typing and retyping successive drafts of the manuscript. Miss Mele was, in addition, most helpful in obtaining necessary materials from the files. I gladly acknowledge my debt to Alna and Elva Kiser for their help with the manuscript and extend my gratitude to Dr. L. E. Burney and David P. Willis for their critical reading of the manuscript and for their suggestions for changes. Finally, I wish to thank Miss Rose Jacobowitz for her expert editorial work in preparing the manuscript for the printer. However, I absolve all of them from responsibility for any remaining errors and for sins of omission as well as of commission. For these and other shortcomings of the book, I alone accept responsibility.

Clyde V. Kiser

Chapter 1

# Elizabeth Milbank Anderson
## Family Background and Her Private Philanthropy
## Before 1905

ELIZABETH MILBANK ANDERSON, daughter of Jeremiah and Elizabeth
Lake Milbank, was born in New York City, 20 December 1850. Her
family heritage extended back into English and early American history; among her forebears and kinsmen were founders of corporations,
builders of railroads, doctors, lawyers, investment bankers and other
business and professional men.

Mrs. Anderson's grandfather, Samuel Milbank (1776–1853),
was born in England at the outbreak of the American Revolution and
came to the United States in 1794.[1] He was the father of twelve children, of whom two, Jeremiah and Samuel, Jr., will be mentioned here.

Jeremiah Milbank (1818–1884) married Elizabeth Lake; they
became the parents of Joseph Milbank (1848–1914) and Elizabeth
Milbank Anderson (1850–1921), the founder of the Milbank Memorial Fund. Samuel Milbank, Jr. (1805–1865) became the father of
Albert J. Milbank (1840–1912), who was the father of Albert G.
Milbank (1873–1949), the long-time adviser to Mrs. Anderson. Albert G. Milbank was the father of Samuel R. Milbank (b. 1906), the
current Chairman of the Board of Directors of the Milbank Memorial
Fund. (See Fig. 1-1.)

The question is often asked as to how the Milbank fortune was
made. There were several sources. The eighteenth century Milbanks
were apparently yeomanry of modest means in England. Samuel, the
pioneer to the United States, became a brewer in New York City. His
son Jeremiah (1818–84) became a wholesale grocer, and Jeremiah's

FIG. 1–1.   Abridged

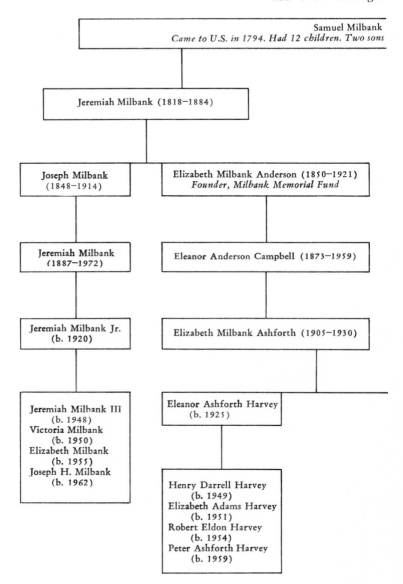

Milbank Family Tree.

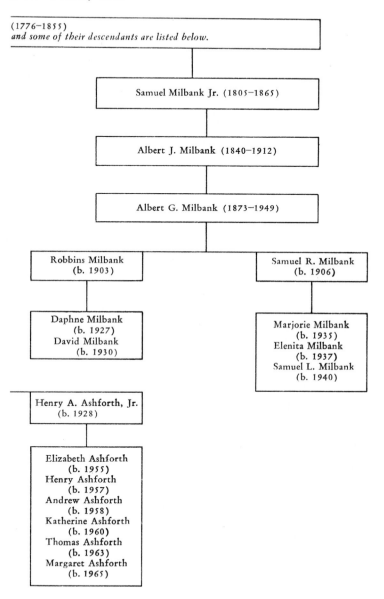

(1776–1855)
*and some of their descendants are listed below.*

Samuel Milbank Jr. (1805–1865)

Albert J. Milbank (1840–1912)

Albert G. Milbank (1873–1949)

Robbins Milbank
(b. 1903)

Samuel R. Milbank
(b. 1906)

Daphne Milbank
(b. 1927)
David Milbank
(b. 1930)

Marjorie Milbank
(b. 1935)
Elenita Milbank
(b. 1937)
Samuel L. Milbank
(b. 1940)

Henry A. Ashforth, Jr.
(b. 1928)

Elizabeth Ashforth
(b. 1955)
Henry Ashforth
(b. 1957)
Andrew Ashforth
(b. 1958)
Katherine Ashforth
(b. 1960)
Thomas Ashforth
(b. 1963)
Margaret Ashforth
(b. 1965)

wife, Elizabeth Lake, was a member of a family of substance in Greenwich, Connecticut.

Jeremiah Milbank proved to be an astute and versatile business man. In an article in *Fortune,* T. A. Wise described the circumstances of the initial encounter of Jeremiah Milbank and Gail Borden:

> In the summer of 1857, Jeremiah Milbank took a fateful train trip. He had been visiting his in-laws in Connecticut. His seat mate on the train back to New York was a Texan who was looking for financial backing to launch a company to produce condensed milk. No one had yet succeeded with canned milk, and Milbank was intrigued. He suggested he might help out if the Texan failed to get the financial backing he expected in New York.

> A little later, the Texan called on Milbank, who promptly put up $50,000, and Gail Borden and Jeremiah Milbank became equal partners in the New York Condensed Milk Co. [It was later renamed the Borden Company.]

> Canned milk was used in great quantities in provisioning the northern armies in the Civil War, and by the end of the war Milbank and Borden were wealthy men.[2]

In 1863 Jeremiah and his son Joseph "led the organizing and financing of the construction of the Chicago, Milwaukee & St. Paul Railway," and in 1864 Jeremiah "opened shop as an investment banker and turned over to a son, Joseph, the management of the wholesale grocery business."[3]

Thus Mrs. Elizabeth Milbank Anderson's father gained his fortune principally from what became Borden's milk, but the wholesale grocery business, railroads, and investment banking also contributed. Her inheritance, the source of gifts and bequests to the Milbank Memorial Fund, was derived from all of these fields.

At least two other accounts suggest a slight deviation from Wise's statement that Jeremiah Milbank helped Gail Borden to *launch* a company to produce condensed milk. These state that Borden had already launched "Eagle Brand Condensed Milk" but was having financial difficulties.

In an article based upon an interview with Albert G. Milbank in 1945, Mary Braggiotti wrote, "He's the grand-nephew of Jeremiah Milbank who, in the 1850's backed Gail Borden's failing Eagle Milk Co. thereby making a fortune when the Company's product became a staple food in the Union Army."[4]

A biography of Gail Borden describes him as a native of Norwich, New York, who went to Texas in 1829. He obtained a land grant from Mexico and was a member of a committee which attempted to appease the "Hotspurs" anxious for secession of Texas from Mexico. However, he was later involved to some extent in the Texas Constitutional Convention of 1836, in the affairs of the Lone Star State, and in its admission to the Union. Borden's education was limited; yet in addition to his rather unfruitful efforts at farming, he had intermittent experience as a teacher, surveyor, and newspaper publisher. He had considerable imagination and the tenacity to hold on to an idea despite difficulties.

His first invention was a "meat biscuit," a loaf composed of concentrates of meat resulting from a special process of cooking. The meat biscuit was to provide protein, in convenient and comparatively nonperishable form, for people such as soldiers, sailors, and travelers, who were deprived of regular food supplies for long periods. Borden was awarded a medal for his meat biscuit at the British Food Fair in 1851. He had already begun manufacture and marketing of the product in Galveston and hoped that recognition from the British Food Fair would increase the sales sufficiently for him to get out of debt and to expand his operations. However, despite expensive and time-consuming trips to northern cities to market the product, the meat biscuit business withered away, and Gail Borden turned his attention to another idea—the possibilities of condensed milk.

According to one biography, a persistent but probably apocryphal story is that Gail Borden first became interested in the idea of condensed milk on his return trip from the British Food Fair in 1851. Traveling on a sailing vessel which carried a few cows to supply fresh milk, he observed the insanitary conditions of the stalls and the small amount of milk available for children.

Whatever the circumstances of Borden's initial interest, he managed to resolve some of the practical problems that had beset previous efforts of more highly educated men to manufacture condensed milk. By 1857 his first real factory had begun operations in Burrville, Connecticut, under the name of Gail Borden, Jr. and Company but unforeseen expenses were great, and Borden's previously described meeting with Jeremiah Milbank in that same year probably saved the enterprise from failure.[5]

On 15 June 1876, Elizabeth Milbank married Colonel Abram Archibald Anderson (1847–1940), portrait painter, rancher, and patron of aviation.[6] His studio, which he had constructed on top of the Beaux Arts Building, 8 West 40th Street, was filled with "rare art works and antiques in a lifetime of adventure and travel . . . Col. Anderson's other art works, including portraits of the late Thomas A. Edison and the late John Wanamaker, lined the wall."[7]

Two children were born of the union. A daughter, Eleanor Anderson Campbell, M.D. (1878–1959), was a physician and founder of the Judson Health Center.[8] A son, Milbank Anderson, died of diphtheria at an early age, a loss which is said to have done much to turn Mrs. Anderson's interests toward preventive medicine.

Although she had been born into a wealthy family, Elizabeth Milbank Anderson was always mindful of the problems of the poor. As a young woman she saw the impact of the Civil War and contributed early to the cause of Negro education. During her lifelong residence in New York City she witnessed epidemics of cholera, typhus, smallpox, diphtheria, and other dread diseases. She beheld the annual floods of immigrants and their crowded living conditions on the Lower East Side.

In 1891 she became interested in the work of Dr. Edward L. Trudeau, a physician who had cured himself of tuberculosis with a revolutionary fresh-air treatment and who wished to demonstrate the worth of this treatment. Mrs. Anderson helped him to establish and maintain the Trudeau Sanitarium and her commitments were later assumed by the Memorial Fund Association. The work of the Trudeau Sanitarium and Research Foundation was continued, after Dr. Trudeau's death, through a final grant, in 1917, which established the Trudeau Foundation.

It is possible that her daughter's interest in medicine, at a time when few women entered this field, helped to encourage Mrs. Anderson's early concern with the cause of higher education for women. At all events, one of her first ventures into public affairs was to become a trustee of Barnard College in 1894. Two years later, in 1896, she provided the funds to erect Milbank Hall, used as an administration building on the Barnard campus at 119th Street. "Still later, in 1903, Mrs. Anderson, realizing that the future of Barnard depended upon the control of sufficient property to permit of expansion, purchased at a cost of a million dollars the three city blocks bounded by 116th and 119th Streets west of Broadway and gave to the College the site which has made its development possible."[9]

Appendix 1 reproduces, almost in full, a contemporary news item from a 1903 issue of *The Sun* concerning Mrs. Anderson's gift to Barnard. The article sheds some light on Mrs. Anderson's personality and interests,[10] portraying her qualities of generosity, reticence, strength of will, and readiness to assert—and to fight for—what she believed to be right.

She was generous in charity and almsgiving but she believed that prevention of poverty can best be attained by improving the conditions of the poor. One of the obvious and concrete conditions that she believed could be improved was that of cleanliness. In 1904, cold-water tenements were the rule on the Lower East Side. Furthermore, the flats were crowded with immigrants from rural areas of Eastern and Southern Europe, some of whom had little acquaintance with bathrooms. In 1904, Mrs. Anderson gave, to the New York Association For Improving the Condition of the Poor, the funds for the erection of the Milbank Public Baths on East 38th Street. According to Winslow, the building that she erected was "so perfect in design and operation that it served as a model for the series of public baths subsequently developed under municipal auspices."[11]

In that same year, her cousin, Albert G. Milbank, became a member of the Board of Directors of the A.I.C.P. Whether or not these two events were related, they helped set the stage for the close cooperation of the Memorial Fund Association and the A.I.C.P. that was to come later. The objectives of the A.I.C.P. apparently coincided with Mrs. Anderson's own philosophy regarding poverty.

Mrs. Anderson also believed strongly in temperance. According to Wise, "Elizabeth Milbank was an energetic, strong-minded woman with a wide range of charitable interests. She donated a library to Greenwich, Connecticut, and three blocks of choice New York City real estate to Barnard College, of which she was a trustee and the largest benefactor at that time. With her brother Joseph she made possible a 'People's Palace' in Jersey City, where the poor could enjoy sports and entertainment—but not hard liquor, which she opposed as much as she favored cleanliness."[12]

Samuel R. Milbank, currently Chairman of the Board of Directors of the Milbank Memorial Fund, has summarized Mrs. Anderson's private benefactions prior to 1905 as follows:

> Long before the Fund existed, Mrs. Anderson was known for her large contributions to agencies and institutions which were undertaking constructive activities in public health, education, and welfare. Numbered among these were The National Committee for Mental Hygiene (now the National Association for Mental Health, Inc.), the Trudeau Sanitarium and Research Foundation for Tuberculosis, Barnard College, and the Association for Improving the Condition of the Poor (later to merge with the Charity Organization Society to form the Community Service Society).
>
> It was the late Albert G. Milbank, her cousin, who advised Mrs. Anderson to organize her benefactions by establishing a foundation, and the policies of the Fund through the years have been based on the experience and views of these two individuals.[13]

Albert G. Milbank has described the circumstances leading to the organization of the Memorial Fund Association as follows:

> Elizabeth Milbank Anderson was one of those rare souls who combined a brilliant mind, a love of humanity, a generous nature, and a keen sense of humor. She was an unquestioned individualist but with a profound sense of her

social obligations. She mistrusted fads and visionary theories as solutions for current problems but the honesty of her mind made it impossible for her to ignore a problem even when its solution called for changes in an established procedure. She was a conservative by inheritance and environment but one who understood that the world does not stand still and that when conditions change the cause of conservatism is best served, not by an unreasoning resistance to any change whatsoever, but rather by a willingness to make reasonable changes, in form and procedure, while preserving the sound principles which, like the eternal verities, persist because they are, in fact, based on truth. . . .

As often happens in human affairs a shattering personal loss had a profound effect upon Mrs. Anderson's attitude toward philanthropy. Her only son died of diphtheria when he was still a little boy. As her brave spirit rose to meet the most crushing blow that Fate could have dealt her, she began to give reasoned direction to her generous impulses which up to that time had been the result of emotional rather than of rational processes.[14]

Mr. Milbank's own role is described elsewhere as follows:

Torn between the desire to help and skepticism of the long-range usefulness of dealing with symptoms after the damage had been done, [Mrs. Elizabeth Milbank Anderson] turned for suggestions to Mr. Albert G. Milbank, her intimate adviser. During the discussion that followed, a plan was evolved for the organization of a charitable corporation with which to explore the possibilities of constructive and preventive treatment of human suffering in contrast to the use of palliative measures which were generally in vogue a third of a century ago. And so, on April 3, 1905, came into being the Milbank Memorial Fund (until 1921 known as the Memorial Fund Association), to commemorate Mrs. Anderson's parents, Jeremiah and Elizabeth Lake Milbank.[15]

## References

[1] Born in Essex County, England, Samuel Milbank was only 18 years old when he left home for the United States. According to information supplied by Jeremiah Milbank (b. 1920), on the transatlantic voyage Samuel Milbank met for the first time the woman whom he was to marry six years later.

[2] T. A. Wise, "How Well-Bred Investors Overthrow a Management," *Fortune* (May 1959): 166.

[3] *Ibid.*, pp. 166 and 168.

[4] Mary Braggiotti, "Service to the Community," *New York Post,* 9 October 1945.

[5] Joe B. Frantz, *Gail Gorden: Dairyman of a Nation* (Norman, Oklahoma: University of Oklahoma Press, 1951).

[6] *The National Cyclopaedia of American Biography*, Vol. 23 (New York: James T. White & Company, 1933), p. 49.

[7] Obituary of Col. Anderson, *New York Herald Tribune,* 1 May 1940. In accordance with his own wish, his funeral was held in this studio.

[8] "Judson Health Center came into being in the early summer month period of 1920, as the result of a very generous offer of Dr. Eleanor A. Campbell. A graduate of the Boston University School of Medicine, and a member of an old New York family whose members had done much to advance health educational and preventive relief work in this country and abroad, Dr. Campbell volunteered her services to Dr. A. Ray Petty, pastor of the Judson Memorial Church, in helping to organize and conduct a community health service in the congested tenement district south of Washington Square," *Measuring the Work of a Health Center,* (New York: The Judson Health Center, 1925), p. 11.

Dr. Campbell had previously (7 April 1904) married John Stewart Tanner, and to this union a daughter, Elizabeth Milbank, was born. After the Tanners were divorced, she married Frederick B. Campbell (1 January 1918) and Elizabeth was adopted by her grandmother under the name Elizabeth Milbank Anderson II. This granddaughter married H. Adams Ashforth in 1923. The Ashforths had two children: Eleanor (b. 1925) and Henry Adams (b. 1928). Eleanor married Eldon Harvey, who has served for many years as President of the Judson Health Center. The Harveys' four children (1949–1959) and the six children of Henry Adams Ashforth are, by direct descent, the great-great-grandchildren of Mrs. Elizabeth Milbank Anderson (information in a personal communication from Mrs. Eldon Harvey, dated 4 May 1973).

[9] C.-E. A. Winslow, "The Living Hand: Elizabeth Milbank Anderson," *The Milbank Memorial Fund: Twenty-fifth Anniversary* (New York: Milbank Memorial Fund, 1930), pp. 12–13.

[10] During 1901–1907 the Dean of Barnard College was Miss Florence Gill, an aunt of the author's wife, Louise Kennedy Kiser. Miss Gill was, therefore, Dean at the time of Mrs. Anderson's gift in 1903.

[11] Winslow, *op. cit.,* p. 13.

[12] T. A. Wise, *op. cit.,* p. 168.

[13] Samuel R. Milbank, "Great American Foundations: 6: Milbank Memorial Fund," *The Observer,* [a Junior League publication] (April 1954): 6.

[14] Albert G. Milbank, "The Relationship of the Milbank Memorial Fund to the Field of Health and the Medical Profession," *The Milbank Memorial Fund Quarterly* 13 (April 1935): 102–103.

[15] *Milbank Memorial Fund: Thirty-Five Years in Review* (New York: Milbank Memorial Fund, 1940), p. 6.

Chapter 2

# The Memorial Fund Association, 1905–1921

IT SEEMS DOUBTFUL that Mrs. Anderson and Mr. Milbank realized
the pioneering nature of their undertaking when they decided, in
1905, to organize the Memorial Fund Association. Only a handful of
foundations were in existence at that time. The Carnegie Institution of
Washington had been started in 1902; the General Education Board
(supported by Rockefeller), in 1903. The Carnegie Hero Fund Commission had been founded in 1904 and the Carnegie Foundation for
the Advancement of Teaching was organized in 1905. Most of the
larger foundations of today were organized after the Fund had come
into existence. The Russell Sage Foundation was to be founded in
1907; the Carnegie Corporation of New York in 1911. The Rockefeller Foundation was organized in 1913.[1] Although the Ford Foundation was formally established in 1936, it did not become active on a
national scale until 1950. The Robert Wood Johnson Foundation was
also incorporated in 1936 but remained relatively inactive until recently.

With the benefit of hindsight, we can see that by the turn of the
century the time was opportune for organizing foundations. The money was available and the needs were great. The last quarter of the nine-
teenth century and the first decade of the twentieth were a period of
great contrasts in economic conditions within the United States—a period of industrial expansion and the accumulation of great fortunes by
a few industrial and commercial leaders and a period of poverty for
workers, especially in the ghettos of large cities. The entrepreneurs
with sufficient capital, knowledge, leadership, and luck could accumu-
late great fortunes because they were not affected by high income tax,

by labor unions, or by much social legislation, such as laws regulating
hours of labor, minimum wages, and employment of children. For
these same reasons, the lot of the laboring classes at the turn of the
century was often one of poverty. The need was also exacerbated by
the poor health conditions of the time. By 1905, visitations of cholera,
yellow fever, and smallpox had been virtually ended, but tuberculosis
was rampant among the poor, and the childhood diseases of dysen-
tery, diphtheria, measles, and whooping cough still took their periodic
toll. Moreover, in the ghettos of large cities, and especially on New
York's Lower East Side, overcrowding was intensified by the annual
addition of many immigrants from Southern and Eastern Europe.

It was, therefore, a fateful day when, on 3 April 1905, the certificate of incorporation of "The Memorial Fund Association," executed
by Edward J. Sheldon, Howard Townsend, Dr. Francis B. Kinnicutt,
George L. Nichols, and Albert G. Milbank, the original Board of
Directors, was filed and recorded.

According to the certificate of incorporation the purposes of the
Memorial Fund Association were:

> To further secular and religious education among all class-
> es; to care for the sick, the young, the aged and disabled;
> to minister to the needs of the poor; to improve the physi-
> cal, mental and moral condition of humanity and generally
> to advance charitable and benevolent objects.
>
> To extend financial or other aid or assistance to such indi-
> viduals, corporations, associations or institutions as are
> now, or may hereafter be, engaged in furthering the pur-
> poses above named, or either of them, and to establish,
> promote, maintain and endow, in whole or in part, any
> such corporations, associations or institutions.

Under the terms of the certificate of incorporation, the Memorial
Fund Association "shall have power to acquire by deed, devise, bequest gift or purchase or otherwise real and personal property, and to
hold, invest, reinvest, manage and dispose of same." Under a Deed of
Trust dated 25 May 1907, Mrs. Anderson "transferred to the Association about three million dollars in securities, to be held in trust, to col-

lect the income therefrom, and after applying $5,000 of such income in each year to the charitable purposes of the trustee, to pay over the balance to the creator of the trust during her lifetime. Upon her death the trust was to cease and the fund to become the absolute property of the Association."

Under an amendment to the Deed of Trust dated 28 October 1913 the Association was given "the power to apply to its charitable purposes so much of the income of the trust property as in the judgment of the Directors was adequate or desirable to accomplish such purposes, and to pay the balance of such income, if any, to Mrs. Anderson."[2]

A brief introduction of the five charter members of the Board may assist in showing why each was chosen and in understanding the nature of the Association's activities during 1905–1921.

As has already been indicated, Albert G. Milbank (1873–1949) was a cousin of Mrs. Anderson. Though she was some 23 years the elder, Mrs. Anderson apparently had for some years consulted her cousin frequently and relied upon his judgment in regard to her investments and charitable activities. He agreed to serve as secretary and treasurer of the Memorial Fund Association at the organizational meeting in 1905. Mr. Milbank took an A.B. degree at Princeton University in 1898. After spending a year on a cattle ranch in New Mexico, he began his career as a lawyer in 1899 with the law firm of Masten & Nichols, whose list of clients included The Borden Company. Mr. Milbank served as Chairman of the Board of Directors of Borden's from 1917 until his death in 1949.[3]

George L. Nichols (1860–1932) was one of the original partners in the law firm Masten & Nichols, attorneys for Borden's and the firm in which Albert G. Milbank began his career as a lawyer. Mr. Nichols was a member of the Board of Directors of Borden's. He was apparently not only a valued friend of the Milbank family but a lifelong professional colleague. His young employee and protégé, Albert G. Milbank, became senior partner in the law firm of Milbank, Tweed, Hope and Webb, when it was created 1 January 1931, by the merger of Masten & Nichols with Murray, Aldrich & Webb.[4]

Edward J. Sheldon (1858–1934), a lawyer and an adviser of Mrs. Elizabeth Milbank Anderson, served as President of the Memorial Fund Association for nearly 25 years (1905–1929) and as a member of the Board of Directors until his death. He took an A.B. degree at Princeton in 1879, received an LL.B. at Columbia University Law School in 1881 and returned to Princeton for an M.A. degree, which he received in 1882. He was a trustee of Princeton University and of Barnard College for many years. For some years, Mr. Sheldon was an attorney of the U.S. Trust Company of New York, which served as the Fund's "Treasurer" throughout most of the Fund's history; he became President of the U.S. Trust Company of New York in 1906.

Francis P. Kinnicutt, M.D. (1846–1913), took an A.B. degree at Harvard in 1868 and an M.D. at Columbia in 1871. He was a physician and professor of clinical medicine at the College of Physicians and Surgeons, Columbia University, from 1893 until his death. Dr. Kinnicutt was consultant physician to many hospitals, including St. Luke's, Woman's, Hospital for Ruptured and Crippled, Babies', and Presbyterian, and served on the Board of the Children's Aid Society[5] to which the Memorial Fund Association later contributed. That he was an esteemed friend of Mrs. Anderson as early as 1892 is attested by the news item from the New York *Sun* (refer to Appendix 1) concerning Mrs. Anderson's gift of land to Barnard College in 1903 and to her earlier philanthropies. In 1892, she had offered to build for Roosevelt Hospital a pavilion to be used as a clinic if Dr. Kinnicutt were to be the first director. Perhaps because of this condition, the offer was eventually declined.

Howard Townsend (1858–1935), a lawyer and friend of Mrs. Anderson, probably was chosen partly because of his interest in tuberculosis. Mr. Townsend took an A.B. degree at Harvard in 1880 and was admitted to the Bar in 1883. He "was engaged for many years in effort to have consumptive poor cared for by the State; was 1st president N.Y. State Hosp. for Consumptives at Ray Brook."[6]

The Memorial Fund Association had neither a staff nor a paid executive director during the sixteen years of its existence. It had no separate headquarters of its own under that name. Within his law office, Albert G. Milbank really served in the triple role of executive director, secretary, and treasurer of the Fund, insofar as the day-to-day affairs were concerned. These included central responsibility for investments and income, for disposition of appeals, and for arrangements for Board meetings. (This statement, of course, is not meant to minimize the work of the other Board members or that of Mrs. Anderson herself. However, Mr. Milbank's affiliation with the law firm and with Borden's facilitated stock transactions and the keeping of records. Banking facilities of the U.S. Trust Company of New York were conveniently available next door to his office.)

Thus Mr. Milbank's own office within the law firm served as headquarters of the Memorial Fund Association. According to Miss Catherine A. Doran, who was employed by Masten & Nichols 7 March 1921, and worked for Mr. Milbank on reorganization of Association affairs, Mr. Milbank had previously set aside a desk for affairs of the Memorial Fund Association and usually assigned a secretary to this work. Miss Doran recalled that there had been frequent letters with the salutation "Dear Lizzie" from Mr. Milbank to Mrs. Anderson. In correspondence and by telephone calls, they discussed not only matters of policy but also specific appeals to be recommended for acceptance or rejection at the next meeting of the Board. Mr. Milbank, furthermore, consulted informally with the members of the Board by letter, by telephone, and at chance meetings.

During this time, Albert G. Milbank's increasing responsibilities with Masten & Nichols and with Borden's made him a very busy man. However, he was often described as a good organizer, one who had the ability to see the fundamentals of a problem quickly and to devise ways of meeting it. Furthermore, once he and Mrs. Anderson had decided upon the formation of the Memorial Fund Association, he had deliberately begun preparing himself for this responsibility.[7]

According to the *Initial Report of the Organization and Development of the Milbank Memorial Fund Since 1905*, prepared for the 11 May 1921 meeting of the Board of Directors, "During the sixteen years of its operation under the name of 'The Memorial Fund Association' the Fund received from Mrs. Elizabeth Milbank Anderson gifts the par value of which amounted to $7,815,175. By her will, Mrs. Anderson left the Fund $1,500,000, thus increasing the entire amount of her gifts, at par value, to a total of $9,315,175." (Refer to Appendix 3.)

The appropriations made by the Memorial Fund Association during the sixteen years 1905–1921 amounted to slightly over 1.5 million dollars. The very first grant made by the Association was one to the Legal Aid Society. A complete listing of the beneficiaries and amounts involved in the grants during 1905–1921 is given in tabular form in Appendix 3, taken directly from a report dated 11 May 1921. As explained in this *Initial Report,* the listing "points to the rather marked tendency to emphasize child welfare and public health work, including mental hygiene. This is more clearly indicated if the appropriations for war relief and war work, made as a result of the great world crisis, are eliminated from consideration. The action of the Board in making this distribution very closely follows the dominant and well known interests of the donor of the funds. Mrs. Anderson, throughout her purposeful life, always gave liberally to relief in a great emergency, although her clear preference was to support organizations interested in child welfare, especially in its preventive aspects, and those engaged in public health and preventive medicine. It is evident, therefore, that the Milbank Fund, while not crystallizing its interests into fixed policies, has shown a clear tendency to devote the major portion of its income to child welfare and public health."[8]

The Association for Improving the Condition of the Poor looms large as a beneficiary of the Memorial Fund Association. It will be recalled that Mrs. Anderson had given a public bath to the city through the A.I.C.P. before the Memorial Fund Association was established. Her cousin was a member of the Board. Thus the A.I.C.P. became a natural channel for grants toward improving the condition of the poor.

In a long letter dated 5 March 1913, addressed to R. Fulton Cutting, President of the New York Association for Improving the Condition of the Poor, Mrs. Anderson indicated her readiness to finance various activities under a Department of Social Welfare which A.I.C.P. had agreed to create. The complete text of this letter is included in the *Initial Report* (Appendix 3). It serves to summarize Mrs. Anderson's interests and to clarify her basic philosophy and attitudes regarding certain social problems and how they should be handled and provides a picture of the donor's first concern with such fundamentals as providing baths, school lunches, public bake shops, medical inspection for school children, clinic facilities, sanitary drinking fountains, clean school rooms, and improved school ventilation. Although some parts of the letter may seem a bit paternalistic—even naive and simplistic—to social and health workers today, Mrs. Anderson's gifts of funds probably did as much as or more than any equivalent public or private expenditures to better conditions on the Lower East Side during the first two decades of the century.

During this period Mrs. Anderson gave to the Children's Aid Society land and buildings in Chappaqua, New York, for the establishment of a convalescent home for children from the poorer areas of New York City. Established in 1912, Chappaqua Home was maintained in part by supporting grants both from Mrs. Anderson and from the Memorial Fund Association. From 1912 until 1922, the Home provided convalescent care for 7,903 children, of diverse backgrounds, who had been referred by hospitals and charitable institutions in the New York City area. "These little patients were convalescing from all sorts and conditions of children's diseases, practically the only limitation being placed on patients convalescing from pulmonary tuberculosis . . . . The institution receives both boys and girls, although there is a necessary age limit of ten years placed on the boys admitted, owing to the fact that the children are all housed in the same building."[9] This project clearly demonstrated both the feasibility and the benefits of convalescent care in a rural environment for children from impoverished urban families. In a larger context, it was a precursor of plans to give children from poor urban families an opportunity for a brief period of rural residence.

Mrs. Anderson's donation of Victoria Apartments to be used as a "Home Hospital" provided a demonstration of the possibility of keeping families intact when a parent contracts tuberculosis.

> The Home Hospital is a new type of institution for the treatment and prevention of tuberculosis, organized by the A.I.C.P. in 1912 as such an experiment, and later continued as a demonstration, to determine the feasibility of treating the patient in his home while at the same time providing proper safeguards for well members of the family, especially the children. The Milbank Memorial Fund was one of the original contributors to this work, pledging $2,000 a year during the experimental stage. Later when the institution was closed as a result of change in the city

administration, the Fund pledged $20,000 a year—one half of the operating cost—to enable the A.I.C.P. to re-establish this work which evidently had made a profound impression upon leading public health authorities and medical experts. . . .

Dr. James Alexander Miller . . . said the Home Hospital had demonstrated two very important things, viz:

1.–That children can be cared for in a family in which there is tuberculosis without danger of infection.

2.–That the parents themselves do as well under Home Hospital treatment as in any sanatorium.[10]

Thus the sixteen years of the Memorial Fund Association helped to prepare the way for the more ambitious programs which were to be undertaken after Mrs. Anderson's death. The initial experience not only provided a test of approaches to specific health problems; it was also a period for identifying and developing leaders for the years to come. Through its support of A.I.C.P. and State Charities Aid Association, in particular, the Association was incidentally preparing such men as Albert G. Milbank, John A. Kingsbury, Bailey B. Burritt, and Homer Folks to play important roles in the future work of the Fund.

It should also be emphasized that the charter members of the Board of Directors helped to put the Association on a firm foundation. In addition to the original Board of five previously mentioned, five others were elected before Mrs. Anderson's death in 1921. Two of these were relatives. Albert J. Milbank, the father of Albert G. Milbank and treasurer of the New York Condensed Milk Company (Borden's),[11] became a Member of the Board and Treasurer of the Memorial Fund Association on 27 May 1907; he served in both capacities until his death 23 May 1912. The other relative was a physician, Dr. Charles M. Cauldwell, who was elected to the Board on 16 January 1914, to replace Dr. Kinnicutt who had died 2 May 1913.

On 29 December 1920, John George Milburn, a lawyer and a trustee of Barnard College, was elected to succeed Dr. Howard Townsend who had resigned.[12] On 17 January 1921, the Board voted to increase its membership to seven. Elected on that date were Elihu Root, one of Mrs. Anderson's lawyers, who had been Secretary of War under McKinley and Secretary of State under Theodore Roosevelt, and

Thomas Cochran, an economist and a partner of the J.P. Morgan Company, who was eventually to urge the Fund into studies of population. A list of past and current members of the Board of Directors of the Milbank Memorial Fund may be found in Appendix 4.

## References

[1] For a list of 100 foundations and trusts organized before 1932, see Eduard C. Lindeman, *Wealth and Culture* (New York: Harcourt, Brace and Company, 1936), pp. 55–57. See also *The Foundation Directory, Edition 4* (New York: Columbia University Press, 1971).

[2] From Minute adopted by the Board of Directors of the Milbank Memorial Fund at a Meeting held 11 May 1921.

See also *The Memorial Fund Association* (a pamphlet containing Deed of Trust dated 27 May 1907 and amendment to Deed of Trust dated 28 October 1913).

[3] See The President's Report to Stockholders and Employees, The Borden Company, Annual Report for 1949, p. 7.

[4] See obituary of George L. Nichols in the *New York Herald-Tribune*, 5 March 1932,

[5] *Who Was Who in America* (Chicago: A.N. Marquis Co., 1942), p. 680.

[6] *Who's Who in New York* (New York City: Who's Who Publications, 1929, p. 1722

[7] A Minute prepared by Board members on the occasion of Mr. Milbank's death and adopted at the meeting of the Board, 21 October 1949, included the following:

> His desire to advise his cousin wisely and to insure the success of the Fund in achieving its humane ends, led Mr. Milbank to study closely the uses to which larger funds could be put in order to give the unfortunate and handicapped the most effective and permanent help. With this object in view he sought the advice of leaders in public health, medicine and welfare, and in turn he became their adviser as well as their intimate and friend. His interest in measures to relieve the unfortunate and his widening experience in this field caused him to be sought after by private and public welfare agencies, and he joined the boards of such agencies as the A.I.C.P., the Welfare Council, and the Community Service Society. Every agency with which he was associated came to rely on his vision and judgment, and in emergencies their leaders always turned to him. In spite of the increasing pressure of other duties, he gave freely of his time and skill to community causes until his last illness brought his part in these activities to a close. . . .

> He could analyze appeals for assistance dispassionately and answer a fool according to his folly but in the end the generosity of his spirit always weighed heavily in the balance of his judgment.

[8] *Milbank Memorial Fund: Initial Report of Its Organization and Development Since 1905* (New York: Milbank Memorial Fund, 1921), p. 5 (hereafter cited as *Initial Report*).

[9] *Ibid.*, p. 15.

[10] *Ibid.*, pp. 22–23.

[11] According to Wise, Mrs. Anderson inherited 25 percent of Borden's stock from her father and entrusted its management to her cousin, Albert J. Milbank. T. A. Wise, "How Well-Bred Investors Overthrow a Management," *Fortune* (May 1959).

[12] According to *Who Was Who,* President William McKinley was taken to Milburn's home in Buffalo after he had been shot by an assassin in 1901. He died in Milburn's home. *Who Was Who in America, Vol. 1, 1897–1942* (Chicago: A. N. Marquis Co., 1942), p. 837.

Chapter 3

# The Tenure of John A. Kingsbury and
# Edgar Sydenstricker, 1922–1936

## Part I: The Health Demonstrations, 1922–1936

ON SEVERAL OCCASIONS in the sixteen years between the founding of the Memorial Fund Association and the death of Mrs. Elizabeth Milbank Anderson on 22 February 1921, she had increased the funds available to the Association. Apparently aware that she did not have long to live, Mrs. Anderson disclosed to Albert G. Milbank and other members of the Board, shortly before her death, her intention to bequeath additional grants in her will. She also expressed a wish to have the Association's name changed to "Milbank Memorial Fund" within one year after her death. To implement her plans, a Special Committee on Organization, consisting of Mr. Sheldon and Mr. Milbank, was appointed at the 17 January 1921 meeting of the Board.

The work of this Committee necessarily assumed a more definite form and greater urgency after Mrs. Anderson's death: Its immediate tasks included preparation of a Minute concerning the death of Mrs. Anderson (Appendix 2) and the legal matters involved in the Association's change of name, which became effective 16 April 1921.

A prophetic step was also taken toward the long-range mission of the organization. The Special Committee arranged for "retaining Mr. John A. Kingsbury as Consultant to make a survey of the work of the Milbank Memorial Fund since its inception, and to prepare an historical summary of its development and operations, together with a classified list of all beneficiaries, to prepare a statement concerning the existing pledges and commitments, to analyze pending appeals, to consult

22

with other foundations and organizations regarding pending and prospective appeals, and to make recommendations as to plan of organization, practice, procedure, forms, etc. both as affecting the management and the contacts with outside organizations, at a fee of $1,250."[1]

Part of Mr. Kingsbury's task was fulfilled by his preparation of the *Initial Report* of the Milbank Memorial Fund for the 11 May 1921 meeting of the Board. This *Report,* mentioned in Chapter 2 and reproduced in part in Appendix 3, contained a historical summary of the organization and a tabular list of its disbursements.

On 7 March 1921, two weeks after the death of Mrs. Anderson, Miss Catherine A. Doran had been engaged to help Mr. Milbank to prepare for the 11 May 1921 meeting of the Board. In this secretarial capacity, she assisted Mr. Kingsbury in preparing the *Initial Report* and in compiling the list of grants made by the Memorial Fund Association during the sixteen years of its existence. Mr. Milbank was so pleased with her work that he offered her a choice: either to remain with him at the law firm of Masten & Nichols or to become the first staff member of the reorganized Milbank Memorial Fund. She decided to join the Fund.

At the 11 May 1921 meeting, the Board adopted the Minute in memory of Mrs. Anderson and formally approved four actions already taken by the Special Committee on Organization: (1) leasing office space at 49 Wall Street, (2) retaining John A. Kingsbury to make a survey of the Fund's work since its inception and to prepare the *Initial Report,* (3) arranging for Mr. Kingsbury to serve as a part-time consultant for one year (from 15 May 1921) and to make recommendations concerning the Fund's future program, and (4) arranging for the services of Miss Catherine A. Doran and further assistance as circumstances should require.

The selection of John A. Kingsbury as consultant to the Fund during the coming year and as advisor on its future program and organization was a natural one. He had prepared the *Initial Report,* and, prior to World War I, he had been General Director of the New York Association for Improving the Condition of the Poor, which had been a major recipient of grants from the Memorial Fund Association.

At a meeting on 22 May 1922, the Board of Directors of the

Milbank Memorial Fund received Mr. Kingsbury's report. It provided an evaluation of the past work of the Memorial Fund Association and recommendations for a future program and praised the judgment of Mrs. Anderson, Mr. Milbank, and the other members of the Board of Directors in emphasizing preventive work rather than simple charity. In particular, the report commended the principles set forth in Mrs. Anderson's letter to the A.I.C.P. in 1913, the success of the A.I.C.P. in implementing these projects, and the effect of some of these projects on city and state policies of health and welfare.

However, the report emphasized that the time had come for the Milbank Memorial Fund to begin its own positive program of disease prevention and health improvement. This program, the report suggested, should be focused upon an important aspect of public health. Specifically, the recommendation was to conduct a demonstration program in the prevention of tuberculosis, and, furthermore, that there be three concurrent demonstrations in different types of communities in New York State: a rural area, a city of medium size, and a metropolitan area.

It is difficult to say who deserves most credit for the initial idea of the New York health demonstrations. Himself a leader in health and welfare, Mr. Kingsbury also enjoyed the benefit of social and professional relations with other leaders in the field. First to be mentioned were three men "he called into council, as an informal group to advise and assist" when he was asked in 1921 to evaluate the past work of the Fund and to appraise the needs and opportunities for future efforts. These were Homer Folks, Secretary of the State Charities Aid Association; Bailey B. Burritt, General Director of the Association for Improving the Condition of the Poor; and Dr. Donald B. Armstrong, Executive Officer of the Community Health and Tuberculosis Demonstration at Framingham, Mass.[2]

In addition, Kingsbury and his associates were acquainted with most or all the other men who were to become charter members of the Technical Board and with most of those who were to become charter members of the Advisory Council. It should be emphasized, however, that there was a recognized precedent for the New York demonstrations: the Commnity Health and Tuberculosis Demonstration initiated in 1917, in Framingham, Massachusetts, by the Metropolitan Life Insurance Company and carried out under the direction of the National Tuberculosis Association.[3]

From the beginning it was agreed that the New York demonstrations should place special emphasis on, but would not be restricted to, tuberculosis control. The continuing health problem of tuberculosis, the Association's past support of efforts at tuberculosis control, and, particularly, a desire to apply the Framingham methods to other types of communities prompted the decision to emphasize tuberculosis control in the project (which was initially called the New York Health and Tuberculosis Demonstrations).

On the other hand, the breadth of talent and interest represented on the Technical Board and Advisory Council afforded a virtual guarantee that the demonstrations would not be restricted to a single disease. These members of the Board and the Council believed that, in the long run, tuberculosis control could most effectively be achieved by integrating such efforts with a comprehensive community program of public health. Thus the "numerous consultations with a representative group of leaders and specialists, resulted in recommendations, subsequently endorsed by the Board of Directors, involving a greater degree of consolidation of the Fund's resources into a distinctive disease prevention and health promotion program, wich special emphasis on tuberculosis control."[4]

Thus at the 22 May 1922 meeting, the Board of Directors appointed Mr. Kingsbury Secretary of the Milbank Memorial Fund, and requested him to proceed with the development of plans for the three demonstration projects.

At this same meeting, the Board of Directors passed two resolutions which not only established two types of advisory bodies to develop and guide the demonstrations but also bestowed two unique and enduring features upon the Fund's structure and activities. These resolutions created the Technical Board and the Advisory Council. The two resolutions were as follows:

> RESOLVED: That the following be asked to serve as members of the Technical Board of the Fund, for the purpose of maturing the plan for the tuberculosis demonstrations, and to submit definite recommendations to the Board

of Directors from time to time with reference to the selection of localities, the designation of operating agencies, and, as the demonstrations progress, to advise with reference to the distribution of functions and to the various operating agencies: . . .

Dr. Hermann M. Biggs, Commissioner of Health, New York State

Mr. Bailey B. Burritt, General Director, New York Association for Improving the Condition of the Poor

Mr. Homer Folks, Secretary, State Charities Aid Association

Dr. James Alexander Miller, President, New York Tuberculosis Association

Dr. Linsly R. Williams, Managing Director, National Tuberculosis Association

Dr. Livingston Farrand, President, Cornell University

Dr. William H. Welch, Dean, School of Hygiene and Public Health, The Johns Hopkins University

Mr. John A. Kingsbury, Secretary, Milbank Memorial Fund

RESOLVED: That the following be asked to accept membership in the Advisory Council for the Tuberculosis Demonstrations, such Council to be called together from time to time or consulted by mail on the initiative of the Board of Directors of the Milbank Memorial Fund or of the Technical Board.

[Those listed included the above-mentioned members of the Technical Board and the following:]

Dr. Donald B. Armstrong, Executive Officer, National Health Council

Dr. Edwin R. Baldwin, Director, Trudeau Foundation

Mr. Cornelius N. Bliss, President, New York Association for Improving the Condition of the Poor

Dr. Lawrason Brown, Medical Director, Trudeau Sanatorium

Mr. George F. Canfield, President, State Charities Aid Association

Dr. Hugh S. Cumming, Surgeon General, United States Public Health Service

Mr. Henry S. Dennison, President, Dennison Manufacturing Co., Framingham, Mass.

Dr. Louis I. Dublin, Statistician, Metropolitan Life Insurance Company

Dr. Haven Emerson, College of Physicians and Surgeons, Columbia University

Dr. Simon Flexner, Director, Rockefeller Institute for Medical Research

Dr. Lee K. Frankel, Third Vice President, Metropolitan Life Insurance Company

Dr. Charles J. Hatfield, Executive Director, Henry Phipps Institute for the Study and Prevention of Tuberculosis, University of Pennsylvania

Dr. L. Emmet Holt, President, National Child Health Association

Dr. Allan K. Krause, Director, Kenneth Dows Foundation for Tuberculosis, Johns Hopkins Hospital

Dr. David R. Lyman, Medical Director, Gaylord Sanatorium, Wallingford, Conn.

Dr. A. J. McLaughlin, Assistant Surgeon General, United States Public Health Service

Dr. T. Mitchell Prudden, Public Health Council, New York State

Professor E. R. A. Seligman, McVicker Professor of Economics, Columbia University

Dr. Theobald Smith, Director, Department of Animal Pathology, Princeton, N.J.

Mr. Fred Stein, New York Tuberculosis Association

Dr. Philip Van Ingen, National Child Hygiene Association

Dr. William Charles White, Medical Director, Tuberculosis League of Pittsburgh

Professor Walter F. Willcox, Cornell University

Dr. C.-E.A. Winslow, Yale University

[and the]

Health Officers of the two cities and the rural county to be selected for the demonstrations.

The organizational meeting of the Advisory Council was not called until 16 November 1922. However, the smaller Technical Board became active immediately.[5] As soon as it had been formally created it submitted and secured passage of the following resolution to collect the demographic data needed for choosing the demonstration areas:

RESOLVED: That steps be taken immediately, in accordance with the suggestion of Dr. Hermann M. Biggs, to make a careful statistical analysis of data, most of which [are] available in the files of the State Department of Health in relation to population, sex, age, race, occupational distribution, etc., and also to collate the essential social data for the upstate cities and counties which would fall within the population range indicated for such tuberculosis demonstrations.[6]

The Health Demonstrations began in Cattaraugus County and Syracuse in 1923 and in New York City in 1924. They have been ably described and evaluated in three volumes by Dr. C.-E. A. Winslow; these are devoted, respectively, to Cattaraugus County, to Syracuse, and to the Bellevue-Yorkville area of New York City.[7]

A general objective of all three demonstrations was to test the possibility of improving public health through more efficient organization and better utilization of health resources. There were, in addition, specific objectives in each of the three areas. Thus, in Cattaraugus County the focus was on the possibilities and potentialities of a county health department and the lessons for other rural counties. In Syracuse, the focus was on the structure and function of a city health department. In the Bellevue-Yorkville area, the focus was on district health organization and ways and means of meeting the health needs in a given city area.

### The Cattaraugus County Demonstration

Since the Cattaraugus County project was the first started and, to some extent, illustrates the general principles and human problems encountered in all three, it will receive particular emphasis here.

In the first place, as soon as the local leaders of Cattaraugus County learned of the possibility of the demonstration, they took steps to encourage the selection of their area. A formal resolution extending an invitation and offering to cooperate was passed by the Board of Supervisors of Cattaraugus County on 12 October 1922. On 16 October 1922, a special meeting of the Cattaraugus County Medical Society unanimously adopted the following resolution:

> Whereas, the Milbank Memorial Fund will initiate and help finance an intensive Health Demonstration in a rural county of New York during the next five years to show what can be accomplished in the prevention of tuberculosis and in promoting the general health and physical vigor of the people,
>
> Therefore, Be It Resolved, that the Cattaraugus Medical Society approve this demonstration and that if Cattaraugus County is selected, it will cooperate in every way that it can to make the demonstration a success.[8]

Cattaraugus County was selected 20 November 1922. Plans for the Demonstration were laid with great care. Homer Folks, Secretary of the Association and a member of the Fund's Technical Board, was well known not only for his deep commitment to health and welfare and for his energy and talents at organization and administration, but also for his sensitivity to human nature and public relations. He counseled his assistants to avoid giving the impression that outside city people were trying to tell the local rural people how the demonstration should be run. It was arranged that the State Charities Aid Association should handle the administrative and public relations aspects.

Since a major purpose of the demonstration was to test the feasibility of tuberculosis control and general health promotion under the aegis of a rural county health department and, conversely, to demonstrate that these goals could be attained by a properly organized rural county health department, as an initial step in meeting the conditions imposed by the planners of the demonstration, a County Department of Health was organized, with headquarters in Olean.

This was in itself a trail-blazing move. Although county departments of health had already been established in other parts of the country,[9] Cattaraugus County was the first rural county in New York State to have a county health department. In effect, the demonstration and the Cattaraugus County Department of Health began life together.

However, it is true that Cattaraugus County was on the verge of having a fully organized health department before the demonstration began. As Winslow stated, the leaders in Cattaraugus "had for some time desired to make a serious attempt to meet the health needs of the people of the County. They had established a county tuberculosis sanatorium in 1916 and in the same year the Olean Chamber of Commerce made the establishment of full-time county health service a part of its program."[10] Perhaps this situation helps to explain the selection of Cattaraugus County as the site for the demonstration.

Whatever the reason, in "January, 1923, the demonstration was formally initiated by the act of the County Board of Supervisors through the creation of a general health district—the first organized county health unit in New York State . . . . A County Board of Health was appointed by the Board of Supervisors, consisting of Mr. John Walrath of Salamanca, president, Mr. William C. Bushnell of Little Valley, Mr. William A. Dusenbury of Olean, Dr. Myron E. Fisher of Delevan and Miss Lilla C. Wheeler of Portville. As no properly qualified local candidates were available, this Board appointed Dr. H. A. Pattison of the National Tuberculosis Association to serve as temporary county health officer until in March, Dr. Leverett D. Bristol, formerly State Commissioner of Health in Maine, was appointed County Health Officer and director of the demonstration, with headquarters at Olean."[11]

Six bureaus were planned: communicable diseases; laboratory diagnosis; tuberculosis; statistical records and reports; maternity, infant, and child hygiene; and health education and publicity. These bureaus were administered by highly competent chiefs. The Bureau of Communicable Diseases was placed directly under Dr. Bristol. The City Laboratory of Olean became the County Laboratory, retaining its director, Dr. Joseph P. Garen. To direct the Bureau of Tuberculosis,

Dr. Stephen A. Douglas of Ohio was employed. The Bureau of Records and Reports was entrusted to the direction of Mr. Fred L. Thompson, who later became director of statistical records in the New York City Department of Health. During the fourth year of the demonstration, the work in maternal, infant, and child health, to which the other Bureaus contributed, was placed in a program under the direction of Dr. Doris Murray. For the work in health education, cooperation was sought and secured from the local schools which, under State law, were responsible for matters and procedures affecting the health of school children.

As has already been stated, the detection, treatment, and prevention of tuberculosis was a primary objective of the demonstration. The work included an intensive case-finding program, provision for medical and nursing care of positive cases, postgraduate training for physicians and nurses and health education for all residents, follow-up service for patients and their families, and the stimulation of maximum use of available sanitaria and rehabilitation services.

The work in maternity, infant, and child health was directed toward "organized health education and specific advisory and remedial medical service for the mother from an early period of pregnancy, at the time of delivery and during post-partum convalescence, and for the child through the period of infancy, preschool and school life."[12]

A Bureau of Public Health Nursing and a Social Service Department met the needs of nursing and social service in all activities of the demonstration. These activities included surveys of nutrition and morbidity, well-baby clinics, school health programs including examinations of tonsils, teeth, and eyes, venereal disease programs, and a host of other services.

For several years, the demonstration had smooth sailing. The internal staff operation appeared to work well. Local political leaders gave the promised cooperation. Not surprisingly, as the end of the demonstration period approached, there was some bickering regarding the extent to which the County should assume the costs of the services.

It was from the Cattaraugus County Medical Society, however, that open hostility erupted. This occurred despite the resolution of welcome and cooperation which the Society had passed in order to bring the demonstration to Cattaraugus County. Winslow described it as follows:

> The first break in cordial relations occurred in September, 1926, when, out of a clear sky and with no warning, the Medical Society passed a resolution criticizing the work of the demonstration. No specific allegations were made and the gravamen of the charges appeared to be failure to consult the Society sufficiently with regard to program and policies. It was apparent that many of the physicians had originally gained the impression that the demonstration was to deal only with tuberculosis and resented its extension into wider fields.[13]

When the County Board of Health learned of the Society's resolution it invited the Medical Society to a meeting of the Board for a frank discussion of the program. The result was a reconciliation. However, on 4 August 1927, the Society passed another resolution:

"That the Cattaraugus County Medical Society go on record as desiring the withdrawal of the Milbank demonstration from this County and opposing any request for the continuation after the termination of this year."[14]

According to Winslow, this second resolution had been prompted by the decision of the Board of Health to request a continuation because the Board felt that it could not carry the full program by the end of 1927.

Whatever the provocation, the Society's resolution provoked an outburst in opposition to it on the part of nurses, staff members of the demonstration, and the health department. Perhaps Reginald M. Atwater, M.D., who became Commissioner of Health for Cattaraugus County in 1927, helped both to allay the opposition of the Medical Society and to encourage the Fund to continue its support a little longer. At all events, the Fund's support was continued throughout seven full years, 1923–1929.

Although he was, naturally, in favor of the Fund's work, Winslow attempted a dispassionate appraisal of the demonstrations. He regarded the eventual opposition of the Medical Society as an understandable reaction. Rightly or wrongly, some of the Society's leaders probably regarded the demonstration as a threat to their economic interests. Also, although the visitors from New York generally tried hard to be friendly and considerate toward the local rural doctors, there may have been some occasion for ruffled feelings.

With regard to the medical results of the demonstration, Winslow correctly emphasized the difficulty of statistical appraisal. For various reasons the counties which had been designated as "controls" were not in fact suitable for this purpose. Although the cause was unknown, the mortality rate from tuberculosis had been lower in Cattaraugus than in the "control" counties for many years prior to the demonstration. However, Winslow cited Sydenstricker's finding, that in Cattaraugus County, but not in the control counties, the observed mortality rate during the demonstration period fell below the trend expected from extrapolation of the pre-demonstration rates. He also cited Dorothy Wiehl's research finding that the infant mortality rate from communicable, respiratory, and digestive diseases had declined more abruptly in Cattaraugus than in the control counties after the demonstration began.[15]

In Winslow's view, however, one of the most telling positive results of the demonstration was the County's readiness, despite the bickering mentioned, to continue the expanded work. Still more important was the subsequent spread of the idea of county departments of health to other rural areas.

### The Syracuse Demonstration

The choice of Syracuse as the area for the health demonstration in a city of medium size followed closely upon the selection of Cattaraugus County for the rural demonstration. According to Winslow, the apparent success of the demonstration in Framingham, Massachusetts, was an important reason for the Fund's decision to work in this field and may have been a particularly powerful stimulus for the Syracuse demonstration. In support of this viewpoint, he cited a statement from the State Charities Aid Association concerning the objectives of the Syracuse demonstration which it helped to administer. Pointing out that in Framingham, a city of some 17,000 at the time its demonstration began, the tuberculosis death rate had been reduced by two-thirds as a result of the intensive five-year program, the statement continued:

> Striking and impressive as were the results of the Framingham demonstration, further demonstrations appeared to be necessary to show that substantially similar results may be secured in other and larger communities varying considerably from Framingham in size and showing variations in social, economic and political constitution. Is it possible, in a large city, to locate and bring under adequate medical and nursing care all cases of tuberculosis and to prevent the occurrence of an appreciable part of the present morbidity and mortality due to communicable diseases? If this is possible, can it be done with what may be considered a reasonable expenditure for the population concerned? In the carrying out of the purposes of the demonstration, what is the most efficient utilization of scientific measures available for the prevention and treatment of disease, and how may they be best applied? How can community forces, both official and voluntary, be best organized for this purpose?[16]

As Winslow himself put it, "The purpose of the health demonstration was to test out the claims of the public health experts on a sufficiently large scale to determine what could actually be done in the way of adequate community health organization, how it could best be done, what it would cost, and what concrete results could be attained."[17]

The three important target areas in the Syracuse demonstration were communicable disease, tuberculosis, and health education. With respect to communicable disease, the demonstration emphasized isolation and quarantine, immunization procedures, and laboratory service. As in Cattaraugus County, the tuberculosis program emphasized case finding, tuberculosis nursing, sanitarium care, and after-care. The problem of health education was attacked at many points: school health service, public health nursing, and various efforts at "carrying the message to the people." Initiated in 1923 and terminated 28 February 1931, the Syracuse demonstration lasted a little over seven years. In his general appraisal Winslow listed ten accomplishments, as follows:

1. The reorganization of the Department of Health under a full-time commissioner, with eleven bureaus of which all but three . . . have full-time heads.

2. The establishment of an unusually sound system of vital statistics and record-keeping . . .

3. The development of a program for the control of tuberculosis which Sir Arthur Newsholme pronounced "the best I have known in any area in America."

4. The coordination of the work . . . in the field of maternal and infant hygiene into a compact and coordinated program of real excellence . . .

5. The coordination of the health program for children in the public and parochial schools . . . , the development of a sound program of health service . . . and an excellent program of health education . . .

6. The combination of specialized nursing services . . . into a single well-organized and well-supervised staff for generalized public health nursing, with special attention to nutrition and mental hygiene. . . .

7. An excellent and effective campaign for immunizing school children and preschool children against diptheria.

8. A well-planned program of popular health instruction conducted by the Bureau of Health Education . . .

9. A demonstration program of visiting teacher service of unique excellence.

10. The organization of a health council and of a strong citizens' committee for the support of the community health program.[18]

Winslow, of course, did not claim that all credit should go to the demonstration for the accomplishments listed. Again there were some difficulties with the County Medical Society, but these were not insurmountable. Perhaps Winslow had this in mind when he stated, "Human nature reacts very naturally in its opposition to new ideas and to new forces coming from without its accustomed experience and local entourage. It is perhaps encouraging that so much progress should have been made with so little active friction."[19]

### The Bellevue-Yorkville Demonstration

The Bellevue-Yorkville demonstration was the last of the three to begin and the last to end. Carried out in the home city of the sponsor (Milbank Memorial Fund), the A.I.C.P., and the State Charities Aid Association, it possessed certain advantages over the other two demonstrations. To a greater extent than the others, the Bellevue-Yorkville demonstration represented a flowering of the three organizations' early interests in the health problems of a metropolitan area.

In fact, the very building which had been given to A.I.C.P. by Mrs. Elizabeth Milbank Anderson in 1904 to house the public baths was repurchased by the Fund in 1924, so that it might be converted into a center for the Bellevue-Yorkville demonstration.

As for professional personnel, there were Kingsbury, Bailey Burritt, Homer Folks, and the host of other public health experts on the Technical Board and on the Advisory Council, most of whom were resident in New York City.

Since the organization of public health work was more advanced in New York City than in Syracuse or in Cattaraugus County the question might well be asked as to why the city was chosen as one of the demonstration areas. One probable cause was the wish of the experts mentioned to test some of their theories in their home city, coupled with their desire to apply the collective wisdom of a demonstration to complex metropolitan health problems that had previously defied solution. By the middle 1920s some of the worst diseases, such as smallpox, typhoid fever, and cholera, had been conquered, but tuberculosis, the communicable children's diseases, and venereal diseases were still very serious health problems. Although the 1924 immigration quota act came into force during the very year in which the Bellevue-Yorkville Health Demonstration officially began, the Lower East Side was still the home of newly arrived immigrants from Southern and Eastern Europe.

The objectives of the Bellevue-Yorkville Health Demonstration have been described by Winslow and Zimand as follows:

1. To apply to a given area known facts about the prevention of disease.
2. To interest the district in the improvement of its health.
3. To further develop, by careful analysis and research, methods of public health administration that are practical and useful in a city of the first class.
4. To supplement existing health agencies, both public and private, to such an extent as to make their facilities reasonably adequate to meet the needs of the population. This implies a health program for the district that, if successful, may be applicable to the whole city and to other urban areas.
5. To integrate the work of the demonstration so thoroughly with the Health Department and other agencies that the gains of the demonstration will be conserved after the demonstration itself is completed.[20]

These same writers also describe the "principles" as follows:

1. The demonstration should be organized on the assumption that official responsibility for health work in this district, as in all others of the city, rests with the Health Department. The demonstration then must very properly function as a supplement and aid of the Health Department, and all the activities of the demonstration should be carried on in accordance with the public health laws, the provisions of the Sanitary Code and the rules and regulations of the Department of Health.
2. An effort should be made genuinely to interest the community in the improvement of its health rather than to superimpose a paternalistic program.
3. The demonstration should undertake to supplement existing agencies in so far as they are not at the moment able to finance a complete program, developing health activities under its own direction only as this seems necessary.
4. The demonstration should have constantly in mind a scientific approach to the method of administration of all activities in the district.
5. Appropriations to both public and private agencies

should be in addition to the amount they are already
spending and such contributions would not permit these
agencies to decrease their present expenditures, the appropriations being made in each case only because the
resources of the agencies are such as to prevent them
from providing an adequate service from their own
funds.

6. The Milbank Memorial Fund will look forward to the
gradual withdrawal of financial support from demonstration projects and the gradual assumption of financial
responsibility therefor by the public and private agencies of the community.[21]

The organization of the project included divisions of "health education and publicity, statistics and records, nursing, child hygiene, tuberculosis, dental hygiene, recreation, and social hygiene. . . ." As in
Cattaraugus County and Syracuse, the central focus was tuberculosis
control. Winslow and Zimand state that "the late Dr. Hermann Biggs
has referred to tuberculosis work as the 'best text a public health program can have'."[22]

As in Syracuse, the Bellevue-Yorkville demonstration succeeded
in avoiding outbreaks of hostility from local medical practitioners
such as had been experienced in Cattaraugus County. However, the
demonstration did not always get full cooperation. One such instance
of this was apparent in the work in syphilis. "In the early years [of
the demonstration], assistance was given to certain venereal disease
clinics of the area, in the interest of improving clinical records and extending social service work. The service proved a real factor in raising
the standards of record keeping and of routine procedure, as well as
in demonstrating to those directly responsible the need for additional
facilities and for enlarged staffs. It was, however, discontinued in
1929, and it the same year the adult venereal disease clinic was closed.
This clinic had been intended primarily as a diagnostic service for
physicians and was abandoned when it appeared that it was being
sought less for this purpose than for actual treatment.[23]

Further evidence of indifference followed "an offer to all the doctors of the area to meet the laboratory expenses of any patients unable
to pay for this service, either wholly or in part. Arrangements were

made by the demonstration with several laboratories to make tests, including blood counts, blood chemistry, urinalysis, examination of skin, tissue, gastric contents, feces, and body fluids, basal metabolism, and blood coagulation tests, and blood typing for transfusion. Unfortunately between May, 1930 and the close of the year, only seventeen doctors availed themselves of this service, and it was accordingly discontinued."[24]

Although some work began in 1924, the Bellevue-Yorkville Demonstration was fully operative for seven years, from 1927 to 1933. The total amount expended on the demonstration was about $900,000. During the period of the demonstration, according to Winslow and Zimand, pulmonary tuberculosis mortality declined about 29 percent, as compared with 4 percent in Manhattan as a whole. The infant mortality rate declined about 22 percent, as compared with 4 percent for Manhattan. Of course, these differences may simply be due to earlier improvement in parts of Manhattan other than Bellevue-Yorkville. Deaths from diphtheria virtually disappeared in the whole of Manhattan, including Bellevue-Yorkville, during the period covered by the demonstration.

Perhaps the chief value of the experience in Bellevue-Yorkville was to demonstrate the feasibility and advantages of district health administration. Dr. John L. Rice, Commissioner of Health of New York City, "showed his support of and cooperation with the demonstration in the strongest manner possible, namely, by taking it over as an activity of his Department, [and] at the tenth annual meeting of the Community Health Council of the demonstration said that without doubt this demonstration has led the way for the other health centers that are now developing in the City."[25]

Finally, it may be appropriate to close with a quotation from former Mayor LaGuardia's Foreword to *Health Under the "El."* Fiorello (Little Flower) H. LaGuardia was elected Mayor of New York City in 1933 and served for three terms, 1934–1945. This thoroughly honest and forthright man was noted for his devotion to community medicine, as those attending the Milbank Annual Conference of 1934 learned at first hand. Harry L. Hopkins, who was just beginning his work in Washington during Roosevelt's first term, was an outstanding participant and the speaker at the Conference banquet.

LaGuardia, learning that Hopkins was attending the Milbank Conference, hastened to the New York Academy of Medicine and agreed to talk at the Luncheon Session. Having explained that he was present because this was the only way of seeing Hopkins[26] (from whom he was trying to get work funds for the City), LaGuardia proceeded to talk extemporaneously, and in a manner that delighted the audience, about problems of health and medical care in New York City.

In the Foreword to *Health Under the "El"* (1937), LaGuardia stated:

> The benefit of the public health measures worked out in Bellevue-Yorkville has not been confined to that district. What was tried out with success in one district, is now being extended to the whole city; what was offered there to thousands the City is now offering to millions. The health center has become the basis of our health program. Nine new health centers are now under construction, or just finished. . . . We will construct at least seven additional health centers. . . .
>
> To the Milbank Memorial Fund, which made possible the additional health work done in this district, the people of this City owe a debt of gratitude.[27]

### Results of the Demonstrations

The Milbank Menorial Fund terminated its support of the demonstration in Cattaraugus County on 31 December 1929 and in Syracuse on 28 February 1931. The effective durations were approximately seven years for each of the areas. Although opposition from the medical societies may have hastened the termination of support, in both areas the demonstrations lasted somewhat longer than was originally planned. Although the Bellevue-Yorkville demonstration was initiated in 1924 and was taken over by the New York City Health Department in 1933, the duration of full operation under Fund support was also about seven years. Having terminated support for the demonstrations in Syracuse and Cattaraugus, the Fund would be able to expand its general research activities. These were to include, from all three demonstration areas, continued collection of data needed for evaluation or general research in specific fields of interest.

This brief his tory of the three demonstrations has attempted to portray their failures as well as their successes. In perspective, perhaps their major success was to demonstrate the practicability of certain ideas of health administration that were then considered novel or unconventional. The Cattaraugus County project showed the feasibility of a rural county health department and a county-wide school health service in the Northeast. The Syracuse project demonstrated the value of a full-time health commissioner in a city of medium size. The Bellevue-Yorkville project proved the practicality of district health organization in a metropolitan area. In each case, the acid test of feasibility was the fact that local governments continued the work, following the essential pattern of the demonstration, after the Milbank Memorial Fund withdrew its support.

The reorganized and enlarged Milbank Memorial Fund was quickly catapulted into national prominence by the demonstrations. They were the Fund's principal activity and accounted for over half its expenditures during the mid-decade of the twenties.[28] During the twenties the Fund continued much of its earlier grant program. Among the outstanding recipients were the Judson Health Center which had been founded and directed by Mrs. Anderson's daughter, Dr. Eleanor Anderson Campbell, the New York Association for Improving the Condition of the Poor, National Committee for Mental Hygiene, American Red Cross, Japanese Relief Fund, State Charities Aid Association, American Public Health Association, and Saranac Laboratory of the Trudeau Foundation. Among grants of $10,000 or more which were initiated after Kingsbury's accession were those for the Milbank Memorial Choir, Princeton University Chapel in Memory of Elizabeth Milbank Anderson, the Committee on the Costs of Medical Care, initial full support of the International Union for the Scientific Investigation of Population Problems, the Henry Phipps Institute of the University of Pennsylvania for research in tuberculosis, the New York Commission on Ventilation, National Tuberculosis Association, International Conference of Social Work, and National Board of Medical Examiners.

## Part II: The Development of Intramural Studies
## and the Division of Research

### *Early Statistical Work at the Fund*

From the very beginning of the health demonstrations, there was a realization of the need for sound statistical procedures in selecting the areas to be studied and in attempting to evaluate the effectiveness of the program. The January 1924 issue of the *Milbank Memorial Fund Quarterly Bulletin* carried, on page 37, the announcement, "A Statistical Advisory Committee has recently been appointed by the chairman of the Advisory Council. It includes Professor Walter F. Willcox [Chairman], Professor Robert E. Chaddock, Dr. Louis I. Dublin, Dr. Otto R. Eichel, Miss Jessamine S. Whitney, Godias J. Drolet and Dr. W. H. Guilfoy."

Pages 21 and 22 of the April 1924 *Quarterly Bulletin* recorded progress of the Committee:

> Following a recommendation of the Statistical Advisory Committee, of which Professor Walter F. Willcox of Cornell University is Chairman, the present and future statistical problems presented by the Demonstrations are receiving careful attention. It is recognized that there must be a minimum of uniform data for both the demonstration and the control areas, but beyond these basic general needs each demonstration unit will be assisted in the development of such statistical service as it should maintain on a permanent basis under its own auspices. . . .
>
> At a recent meeting of the Statistical Advisory Committee, it was recommended that a statistician be engaged to assist the operating agencies in developing under local auspices in the demonstration areas, such statistical services as are necessary to the success of the entire project. Through arrangements with the National Tuberculosis Association, Miss Jessamine S. Whitney, statistician of that organization and a member of the advisory committee, has been granted a temporary leave of absence to accept this appointment. Miss Whitney has completed preliminary field studies and has outlined a program of statistical serv-

ices necessary to measure the progress of the demonstrations and to appraise their ultimate results.

According to the Fund's records, Jessamine S. Whitney was employed 17 March 1924 as "statistical adviser—health demonstrations." She resigned from this position 1 February 1925.

One of the developments "under local auspices" was announced on page 22 of the July 1924 *Quarterly Bulletin*. "In Syracuse there had been no definite statistical organization for the demonstration as a whole, each division doing some statistical work along its own lines; including, of course, the routine statistical work done by the City Department of Health. On June first, Miss Mary V. Dempsey was appointed Statistician of the Demonstration. She will be attached to the office of the Commissioner of Health and will assist all the cooperating agencies in their statistical work. Miss Dempsey was formerly Statistician for the American Child Health Demonstration at Fargo, North Dakota, and comes to the work in Syracuse with a very intimate knowledge of the statistical needs of a demonstration."

These paragraphs suggest that, although the planners of the demonstration were aware of the desirability of evaluating the projects from the beginning and, although they took some preparatory steps, they apparently did not realize at first the enormity and the complexity of such a problem. There seemed to be a belief that if "control counties" were designated, the job of testing the work in Cattaraugus would be a relatively simple matter. Certainly there is no evidence on record that the early planners envisaged the future possibility of a Division of Research in the Fund to evaluate the work of the demonstrations.

Whatever the truth of the situation, the activities of the Statistical Advisory Committee do suggest a groping toward stronger statistical control of the demonstrations. Fortunately, among the members of the Advisory Council was Dr. Hugh Cumming, Surgeon General of the United States Public Health Service. Late in 1925, through the cooperation of Dr. Cumming, Edgar Sydenstricker, Public Health Statistician of the United States Public Health Service, was appointed Statistical Consultant of the Milbank Memorial Fund and was specifically assigned to make a survey of the statistical recording systems of the New York Health Demonstrations.[29]

## Impact of Sydenstricker's Work

Sydenstricker's first appointment to the Fund was as a temporary, part-time consultant, his task that of examining the statistical aspects of the three health demonstrations. At his suggestion two of his associates in Geneva, Dorothy G. Wiehl and Jean Downes, were also appointed as temporary research associates of the Fund. Dorothy Wiehl had been a member of the U.S.P.H.S. staff prior to her service in Geneva and had worked with Sydenstricker and Goldberger on pellagra studies in the South.

In following their mandate, Sydenstricker, Wiehl, and Downes were first concerned with the statistical aspects of the three demonstrations. Although they had arrived too late on the scene to help with the original statistical plans, they were able in some instances to assist in improving the methods of data collection. They were also able to help in planning certain studies (particularly in the Bellevue-Yorkville area) that were initiated after their arrival at the Fund.

The fact that Sydenstricker and his associates arrived at the Fund after the demonstrations were well under way perhaps afforded them the advantage of approaching their tasks of evaluation with more objectivity than would have been possible for Kingsbury, Folks, or Burritt. Furthermore, their training as statisticians rather than as social workers had given them the skills required for objective evaluation. It must be emphasized that when Sydenstricker, Wiehl, and Downes came to the Fund in 1926 they brought a "new look." Thereafter, the Fund's operation was to be conditioned not only by the humanistic warmth of the social worker but also by the "hard look" of the statistician.

The Fund's 1926 Annual Report carried Sydenstricker's article "The Measurement of Results of Public Health Work: An Introductory Discussion." This did not attempt to supply indices of effectiveness of the demonstrations but instead discussed the complexity of the problems of measurement and emphasized the necessity of planning the evaluation as part and parcel of an experiment or demonstration. "Measurement of results of public health work is not something that can be done by one who is wholly detached from the work, or after the work has progressed to the point when an evaluation is desirable. The principles underlying measurement and the methods by which it is to be accomplished partake of the very essence of the work itself. They are the basis of inductive reasoning, of scientific procedure, of efficient practice. Upon them and by them clarity in objective is made possible, the ways and means of doing what we set out to do are rendered sound, and results are made satisfying. This is but another way of saying that if we plan and execute our work well, we shall have at hand the basic data and the conditions for proper measurement."[30]

This article was shortly followed by one published in the March 1928 *Proceedings of the American Statistical Association,* "The Statistical Evaluation of the Results of Social Experiments in Public Health." In this instance, Sydenstricker utilized the control counties designated by the planners of the Cattaraugus County demonstration. The planners had selected Jefferson, Steuben, and Chatauqua counties as controls; the last-named adjoined Cattaraugus, and the others were nearby.

As a first step in his analysis, Sydenstricker compared the pre-demonstration mortality rates and showed that, as early as 1900, tuberculosis mortality rates had been lower in Cattaraugus County than in the control counties and that the pre-demonstration decline (1900–1922) had been less steep than in the control counties. As has already been described, however, only in Cattaraugus County did the actual mortality rates for the demonstration period (1922–1927) fall below the "expected" rates provided by extension of the straight lines fitted to the 1900–1922 series. Although he interpreted this as favorable to the work of the demonstration, he issued another warning similar to that previously cited: "Except in rare instances, it will be possible to evaluate statistically the results of social experiments only when proper facilities for measurement are provided as an essential part of the experiment itself. This means that a social experiment ought to be 'set up' on scientific principles, that is, planned, carried out, and observed in such a way as to permit evaluation of the extent to which its objectives are attained."[31]

Sydenstricker's research associates followed his lead in hard-headed analyses. In her article "Infant Mortality in Cattaraugus

County," published in January 1928, Dorothy G. Wiehl adduced data indicating declines in the infant mortality rate during the demonstration period. "But the fact that a decline in deaths of infants took place at this time does not establish what factors brought about this decline."[32] Both Wiehl and Downes carried out studies on the need for accurate official statistics and especially for correction of rates for residence.[33]

Kingsbury and Sydenstricker made an effective team. Kingsbury was the head but he relied heavily on Sydenstricker for technical advice and for advice on matters of policy. Both men were intensely interested in problems of public health and especially in problems of medical care. Sydenstricker attended most of the meetings of the Technical Board and of the Board of Directors. He won the respect and admiration of members of both groups and was well known and liked by the more numerous members of the Advisory Council.

It is, therefore, not surprising that Sydenstricker's temporary appointment as consultant developed into a permanent affiliation. With the encouragement and backing of A. G. Milbank, John A. Kingsbury, and the members of the Board of Directors, Sydenstricker developed plans for a Division of Research within the Fund. The Division was formally organized in 1928, with Sydenstricker as its chief.

In accordance with his philosophy of a multidisciplinary approach to public health problems, Sydenstricker proceeded to add representatives from several fields. Frank W. Notestein joined the staff in October 1928 in order to help initiate the Fund's work in population.[34] Marian G. Randall, R.N., became a staff member on 1 September 1929 in order to make a series of studies of public health nursing in Cattaraugus County, Syracuse, and other areas. On 15 October 1931, the present writer came to the Fund as a Fellow to work with Notestein. Regine K. Stix, M.D., joined in 1932 to assist in the Fund's emerging studies of family planning. Margaret Witter Barnard, M.D., who had worked in the Bellevue-Yorkville demonstration, became a part-time employee of the Fund in 1932, to continue her studies of tuberculosis. Ralph E. Wheeler, M.D., who had worked in the Cattaraugus County demonstration, also came to the Fund in 1932 to analyze data he had collected on whooping cough and various types of adult illness. In 1933, I. S. Falk, who had previously been Associate

Director of Research for the Committee on the Costs of Medical Care, joined the Fund's staff to collate factual materials on health insurance and medical care.

The change from a primary focus on health demonstrations to the activities of a Division of Research was paralleled by corresponding changes in the nature and function of the Technical Board, the Advisory Council, the Annual Conferences, and the *Milbank Memorial Fund Quarterly Bulletin*. All of these agencies and instruments had been created principally for the planning or conduct of the demonstrations. The original Technical Board had been composed of those few (the Secretary of the Fund among them) who had developed the idea of the demonstrations. As a small group meeting frequently with the Secretary, they had exercised great influence. The advice and counsel of the Technical Board was readily available to the Secretary. Through the Secretary, the Technical Board had made recommendations to the Board of Directors not only on matters pertaining to the demonstrations but also on appeals for grants. As a result of the change in direction and structure, the value of the original type of expertise provided by the Technical Board declined. The technical staff employed after the creation of the Division of Research supplied the type of expertise required for the Fund's new research activities. The role of the Technical Board thereafter tended to become that of an advisory body.

The Advisory Council had orginally been created as a forum for hearing and passing judgment upon annual or periodic progress reports on the demonstrations. With the termination of the demonstrations, this purpose of the Advisory Council ceased to exist, and its members adopted a different role. The Annual Conferences were continued, and each year many of the same people appeared, together with new and different faces, because invitations were now issued to individuals rather than to members of an Advisory Council.

Similarly, although the demonstrations provided data for research and conference topics for several years after their termination, the nature of the Conferences changed markedly. Prior to 1932, the Annual Conferences were devoted to short progress reports and discussion concerning the demonstrations. In 1932, the format was changed to round-table discussions to which appropriate specialists were invited. There were, in 1932, five round tables devoted, respectively, to city health centers, education of health personnel, tuberculosis in children, public health nursing, and population.

Finally, after Sydenstricker's arrival the *Milbank Memorial Fund Quarterly Bulletin* changed quickly from a small house organ, devoted primarily to the work of the demonstrations, to a scientific journal of public health and demography with a modest but worldwide circulation.[35]

The period of the early thirties was notable in the history of the Fund. The staff reached its maximum size of some 40 people,[36] and research interests became diversified.

To a considerable extent the economic and political climate of the depression years—the New Deal era—influenced the Fund's affairs. Concern over unemployment led Thomas Cochran, one of the members of the Board, to insist upon the Fund's commencing studies of population and contraception.[37] Having made a substantial grant to New York City for financing local work projects for the unemployed, the Fund in 1932–1933 received an invitation to utilize some "white collar" help for health surveys. Accordingly, plans were made to collect data on health, morbidity, and fertility in relation to changes in employment and income in selected areas of Harlem and Brooklyn in 1933. Shortly thereafter, at the invitation of the U.S.P.H.S., the Fund assumed responsibility for a somewhat similar "Health and Depression Survey" in selected poverty areas of ten cities. G. St. J. Perrott was employed to administer the latter project, which provided something of a proving ground for the U.S.P.H.S.-sponsored National Health Survey of 1935–1936. With funds from W.P.A., Perrott served as administrator of the National Health Survey and later became Director of the Division of Public Health Methods of the U.S.P.H.S.

## Part III: The Retirement of John A. Kingsbury and the Accession of Edgar Sydenstricker as Scientific Director

Although the economic depression served to emphasize the need for better health services, interest in this subject had nevertheless been marked during the prosperous twenties. The Committee on the Costs of Medical Care was organized in 1927, during the Coolidge administration. In the words of the Chairman, Ray Lyman Wilbur, M.D., who was then Secretary of the Interior, "The Committee on the Costs of Medical Care has been created to study a problem which, according to the Secretary of the American Medical Association, is the one great outstanding question before the medical profession today. This, says Secretary [of the A.M.A.] Olin West, is 'the delivery of adequate, scientific medical service to all the people, rich and poor, at a cost which can be reasonably met by them in their respective stations in life'."[38]

The Committee consisted of some fifteen private practitioners of medicine, six people in public health (George H. Bigelow, Herman N. Bundesen, Haven Emerson, Elizabeth Fox,[39] Edgar Sydenstricker, and C.-E. A. Winslow), six representing institutions and special interests (including Lee K. Frankel, of the Metropolitan Life Insurance Company, and Olin West, M.D., of the A.M.A.), five economists (including Michael M. Davis and Wesley C. Mitchell), and eleven from "the public" (including Chellis A. Austin, Homer Folks, Ray Lyman Wilbur, and Matthew Woll).

The research staff included Harry M. Moore as Director of Study, I. S. Falk as Associate Director, and, among the analysts, Niles Carpenter, Hugh Carter, Margaret C. Klem, C. Rufus Rorem, and Nathan Sinai. As described by the Chairman, "The Committee's work is assisted financially not only by the medical profession, but by several of the foundations interested in the advancement of knowledge and the improvement of the people's health. The support of the Carnegie Corporation, the Milbank Memorial Fund, the Russell Sage Foundation, and the Twentieth Century Fund has made possible the inauguration of the Committee's five-year program."[40] Thus, in addition to its financial support, the Fund was represented on the Committee by a staff executive (Sydenstricker), a member of the Board (Austin), a member of the Technical Board (Folks), and by several members of the Advisory Council (Emerson, Frankel, and Winslow).

Both Kingsbury and Sydenstricker were greatly interested in problems of medical care. Furthemore, although a few physicians on the Technical Board and Advisory Council might have been termed conservative in matters of medical care, most of them at least favored the collection of basic data on this particular problem. The Board of Directors endorsed this point of view. With termination of the demonstrations, it was natural for the Fund to support and participate in exploration of a problem that appeared to be of crucial importance.

During the early thirties, the problem of medical care costs and the work of the Committee received much attention at the annual conferences and at the Technical Board meetings. At the dinner session of the 1932 Conference, Albert G. Milbank spoke on "Socialized Capitalism,"[41] and the guest speaker, Dr. Ray Lyman Wilbur, Secretary of the Interior and Chairman of the Committee on the Costs of Medical Care, delivered an address on the economics of public health and medical care. He presented some of the Committee's chief findings.

By 19 May 1932, the Milbank Memorial Fund had appropriated a total of $260,000 toward the research activities of the Committee, which had been directed by Drs. Harry M. Moore and I. S. Falk. At the meeting of the Technical Board on that date, the minutes attest that Dr. C.-E. A. Winslow, Vice Chairman of the General Committee and Chairman of the Executive Committee, described the research as follows:

1. Surveys of data showing the incidence of diseases and disabilities requiring medical services and of generally existing facilities for dealing with them;
2. Studies on the cost to the family of medical services and the return accruing to the physician and other agents furnishing such services; and
3. Analyses of specially organized facilities for medical care now serving particular groups of the population.

The Committee's final report, *Medical Care for the American People*, appeared in November 1932. The five principal recommendations,[42] approved by the majority of the Committee, were as follows:

Recommendation 1.—The Committee recommends that medical service, both preventive and therapeutic, should be furnished largely by organized groups of physicians, dentists, nurses, pharmacists, and other associated personnel. Such groups should be organized, preferably around a hospital, for rendering complete home, office, and hospital care.

Recommendation 2.–The Committee recommends the extension of all basic public health services—whether provided by governmental or non-governmental agencies—so that they will be available to the entire population according to its needs. Primarily this extension requires increased financial support for official health departments and full-time trained health officers and members of their staffs whose tenure is dependent only upon professional and administrative competence.

Recommendation 3.–The Committee recommends that the costs of medical care be placed on a group payment basis, through the use of insurance, through the use of taxation, or through the use of both these methods. This is not meant to preclude the continuation of medical service provided on an individual fee basis for those who prefer the present method. Cash benefits, *i.e.*, compensation for wage-loss due to illness, if and when provided, should be separate and distinct from medical services.

Recommendation 4.–The Committee recommends that the study, evaluation, and coordination of medical service be considered important functions for every state and local community, that agencies be formed to exercise these functions, and that the coordination of rural and urban services receive special attention.

Recommendation 5.–The Committee makes the following recommendations in the field of professional education: (A) That the training of physicians give increasing emphasis to the teaching of health and the prevention of disease; that more effective efforts be made to provide trained health officers; and the social aspects of medical practice be given greater attention; that specialties be restricted to those specially qualified; and that postgraduate educational opportunities be increased; (B) that dental students be given a broader educational background; (C) that pharmaceutical education place more stress on the pharmacist's responsibilities and opportunities for public service; (D) that nursing education be thoroughly remoulded to

provide well-educated and well-qualified registered nurses;
(E) that less thoroughly trained but competent nursing
aides or attendants be provided; (F) that adequate training
for nurse-midwives be provided; and (G) that opportunities be offered for the systematic training of hospital and
clinic administrators.

In view of the Committee's diverse composition, it is not surprising that these recommendations were not approved unanimously. The
final report, therefore, contained minority reports and lists of recommendations. The latter took particular exception to the majority recommendations regarding the organization of medical services and
methods of payment for services. On page 170, the minority recommended "that government competition in the practice of medicine be
discontinued" and, on page 176, "that the corporate practice of medicine, financed through intermediary agencies, be vigorously and per-
sistently opposed."

However, the minority reports did support many of the specific
recommendations of the majority report. On page 152, for example,
appears the statement, "We are in full and hearty accord with the majority in its recommendations for 'The Strengthening of Public Health
Services' and 'Basic Educational Improvements,' and we agree to
some extent with the pronouncements of the Committee in respect to
coordination of medical services."

The last page of the Committee's final report carries Sydenstricker's statement, "As a member of the Committee, I regret that I cannot
see my way clear to sign the final report of the Committee for the reason that the recommendations do not, in my opinion, deal adequately
with the fundamental economic question which the Committee was
formed primarily to study and consider."

The Minutes of the Meeting of the Technical Board on 18 January 1933, two months after the publication date of the Committee's
final report, clarify to some extent Sydenstricker's reluctance to sign
the report:

> The ensuing discussion revealed that the members of
> the Technical Board generally disagreed with the recom-

mendations of the Committee on the Costs of Medical
Care, as set forth in its final report. They agreed, however,
that the Committee had collected much valuable factual
data which with other available material constituted a basis
for further profitable study. This material, Mr. Sydenstricker said, bears (a) upon what medical care people
now receive; (b) upon what people now pay for that care;
and (c) upon what care people need. It includes also surveys of existing schemes for distributing such care. But, in
attempting to compose divergent interpretations of this material into unanimous recommendations, the Committee
had not given expression in its report to recommendations
which were warranted by an impartial analysis of the facts
which it had collected, members of the Technical Board
concluded. They believed that these facts and experiences
might profitably be further studied by the Fund's own staff
under the direction of Mr. Sydenstricker and with the advice and counsel of the Technical Board. Mr. Sydenstricker
said that actuarial material, throwing light upon the
amount of sickness, and of hospitalization and treatments
of various kinds required, would need to be sought further.

The Fund's *Annual Reports* for the years 1932 and 1933 also describe inadequacies perceived in the Committee's work.

Thus no definite comprehensive plan on a nation-wide
or even state-wide basis came out of the five years of study
and deliberation. Although the majority group of the Committee proposed the development of one or more non-profit
"community medical centers" in every city of approximately 15,000 population or more, no program for the establishment of such centers was outlined or proposed.[43]
The failure of the Committee on the Costs of Medical
Care to propose a definite and comprehensive program as a
solution for the conditions revealed by the researches of
the staff, led the Fund to undertake a further study of the
problem. Early in 1933, Dr. I. S. Falk, who had served as
associate director in charge of the research staff of the
Committee, joined the Fund's staff to undertake, in collab-

oration with Mr. Edgar Sydenstricker, further studies directed toward the solution of the problems which the Committee had left unsolved. This study deals primarily with
two economic phases of the problem of medical care. One
is the distribution of the costs of medical care over the
large majority of the population which is able to pay for
medical care but unable to budget emergency costs. The
other is the prompt and adequate remuneration of physicians and others who render medical care. Although economic phases are the main subjects of this inquiry, the relationship of medical care to public medical service and
public health is also being given emphasis in the
study. . . .

The Fund's studies may be divided into three phases.
The first is a review of existing conditions and a resumé of
deficiencies in the medical care of the population. The second is a critical appraisal of various remedies, including
voluntary experiments conducted in this country, medical
practices under Workmen's Compensation Laws, and the
experience of health and sickness insurance systems in European countries. The third will be an attempt, in collaboration with thoughtful physicians, social workers, sanitari-
ans, economists, and others, to propose a statewide system
of medical care.[44]

In describing plans for a round table on medical care at the 1933
Annual Conference (to be held 15–16 March), Mr. Sydenstricker
said that the Fund's technical staff had tentatively defined three postu-
lates, which it deemed fundamental for any method of providing medical care:

1.–That provision for medical care of all the population is
   a measure essential to the maintenance of the health of
   the nation.
2.–That any method must take into consideration the facts:
   (a) That there is a great inequality among the people,
   under our economic system, of ability to purchase medical care; and
   (b) That in the great majority of instances, sickness is an
   unpredictable event and constitutes a financial emergency.

3.—That those who render medical care should be adequately and properly paid.[45]

Shortly after the 1933 Annual Conference, at a meeting of the Technical Board on 15 June 1933, "Mr. Sydenstricker said that the procedure which the Fund's staff was purposing [*sic*] to follow in further exploring its health insurance studies were to publish (a) a summary of the findings of the Committee on the Costs of Medical Care which Dr. Falk had under preparation; (b) an appraisal of the facilities at present available for meeting the requirements indicated in the Committee's Report; and (c) a critical analysis of the experience of other countries in their attempts to offer adequate medical care to groups within their populations. These inquiries, it is anticipated, will be made the basis for the formulation of recommendations for the institution of a health insurance scheme in a political unit of government in this country, preferably a state."[46]

## Circumstances of John Kingsbury's Retirement

No record of dissent can be found, in either the meetings of the Technical Board or the Board of Directors, to Sydenstricker's emphasis on this fact-finding approach toward problems of medical care.

Sydenstricker, surely no less dedicated a man than Kingsbury, chose to deal with the problems as a scientist rather than an activist. Evidently realizing that the topic was "charged with emotional dynamite," he wanted first to collect and analyze objective data that would be needed for guiding efforts at reform.[47]

Kingsbury's philosophy, on the other hand, was that of a social worker, an activist, and a reformer. He had a high regard for Sydenstricker's scientific approach and placed considerable reliance upon it. However, Kingsbury was impatient to get reforms started, and it was in relation to some of his activities that objections emerged and grew.

During the late summer of 1932, Kingsbury and Sir Arthur Newsholme traveled together through the U.S.S.R. to observe the operation of health agencies and systems of medical care. Their book, *Red Medicine*, published in 1933, gave a generally glowing account of medical conditions in the U.S.S.R., although it also contained many comments critical of conditions existing there.[48] At the time of its publication, the book must have antagonized some Americans of conservative views, among whom may have been members of the Technical Board and Board of Directors.

In March 1933, Franklin D. Roosevelt began his first term as President of the United States. Two men who had been close to the work of the Milbank Memorial Fund eventually followed him from Albany to Washington. One of these was Harry L. Hopkins, Kingsbury's former protégé at the A.I.C.P., who had been head of the New York State Temporary Emergency Relief Administration and was to become head of the W.P.A. as well as one of the President's closest advisors. The other was was Thomas Parran, who had been a member of the Fund's Technical Board and Commissioner of Health of New York State and was to serve as Surgeon General of the United States Public Health Service from 1936 to 1948.

During his tenure as Governor of New York, Roosevelt had known Kingsbury and was well acquainted with the Fund's work in health. Moreover, he had appointed Kingsbury to membership on The New York State Health Commission for 1930–1932. Kingsbury quickly recognized the possibilities for greater reforms in the health field that Roosevelt's election might afford and his own—and the Fund's—potential contributions to such reforms on a national scale.

At the 2 February 1933 meeting of the Technical Board, the guest speaker, Harry L. Hopkins, "sketched briefly the problem confronted by T.E.R.A. [Temporary Emergency Relief Administration of New York State] and other groups administering public and private funds in the relief of distress occasioned by the economic depression. He said that there were between 12,000,000 and 13,000,000 wage earners unemployed in the United States, with about 30,000,000 of the population affected directly by unemployment. Approximately 1,750,000 wage earners are unemployed at present in New York State." The need for a medical relief program was also discussed. "Dr. Parran . . . presented a memorandum outlining a tentative proposal [that he had prepared for New York State]. Dr. Parran's plan proposed the establishment of a medical division of the Temporary Emergency Relief Administration in charge of a staff member of the [N.Y.] State Department of Health."[49]

At the 18 January 1934 meeting of the Technical Board, "Mr.

Kingsbury then referred to the editorial statement, 'Health Plan for the Nation,' published in the October [1933] number of the Fund's *Quarterly Bulletin*, which had been brought to the attention of President Roosevelt. Mr. Kingsbury said that he had received a letter from the President expressing interest, requesting Mr. Kingsbury to confer with Secretary [Harold W.] Ickes, Secretary [Frances] Perkins, and the head of hte Public Health Service [Cumming], and stating that he thought he might be ready to take up the question of public health from a national point of view next winter. In response to this request, Mr. Kingsbury and Mr. Sydenstricker last week called upon Secretary Ickes, Secretary Perkins, Surgeon General Cumming, Mr. Harry Hopkins and others . . . .

"Mr. Kingsbury stated that he expected to make a report to the President on his Conferences with Secretary Ickes, Secretary Perkins and the Surgeon General and to recommend that the President designate the heads of the departments concerned, to serve with a group of technical and other experts in the formulation of a plan for his consideration. This proposal appeared to meet with the approval of all present."[50]

However, several members of the Board felt a growing uneasiness about the Secretary's activities. At the 14 June 1934 meeting, Dr. James Alexander Miller "raised the question as to whether an attempt should not now be made by the Technical Board to appraise the Fund's program of activities. Mr. Kingsbury concurred in this, but . . . said that he would like . . . to make a statement to the Technical Board concerning administrative relationships, particularly the relation of the Technical Board to the staff of the Fund. He said it had come to his attention that some members of the Technical Board had expressed criticism of the staff and particularly of the Secretary. He understood it had been stated that the Secretary of the Fund had not really given the Technical Board opportunity for full and free discussion; that the emphasis of certain features of the program had been shifted without full consideration by the Technical Board . . . . "[51]

At the 18 October 1934 meeting, Albert G. Milbank announced that, during Mr. Kingsbury's absence abroad, he had complied with the request of the Executive Director of the President's Committee on Economic Security to have Mr. Sydenstricker and Dr. Falk assist in its study of programs of medical care and public health. He stated that he was heartily in favor of the Fund's collaboration with the President's Committee. He thought it would be better, however, for Mr. Sydenstricker and Dr. Falk not to serve officially as members of the Committee's Technical Staff but to give whatever voluntary aid they could.[52]

At the 6 December 1934 meeting of the Technical Board, "Dr. [James Alexander] Miller expressed the opinion it was extremely important that the Fund move most carefully, especially in the matter of outside professional participation and of cooperation in these activities of the Fund. He emphasized that the Fund is committed to both fields [(a) exploitation of experience accumulated in the health demonstrations and (b) study of health insurance systems] and should be most careful and thoughtful in future work to make the Fund's activities most effective."

At this same meeting even Homer Folks, who had worked closely with Kingsbury for many years, complained that he was not at all clear as to precisely what was covered or what was meant by [the Fund's current] activities listed under the general subject of Economics, and particularly under the subhead, Economic Aspects of Medical Care. He said he knew, of course, that Mr. Sydenstricker and Dr. Falk had been loaned to the President's Committee on Economic Security, but that his only acquaintance with the actual results of the studies being conducted by the staff reached him through an Advisory Committee of the President's Committee rather than through the Technical Board of the Fund.

"As a second point, Mr. Folks said he was disturbed because it seemed, in going into the field of medical economics, the Fund was spreading its interests over a new and broad field. He thought there was still so much to be done in public health that he questioned the wisdom of attempting to spread the limited resources of the Fund over a new field."

In regard to the first point, Mr. Sydenstricker explained that he and Dr. Falk had simply been "loaned" to the President's Committee; no officers of the Fund nor members of the Technical Board had any responsibility for the materials which he and Dr. Falk were developing for the President's Committee.

As to the second point, Dr. Livingston Farrand, Chairman of the

Technical Board, expressed his confidence "that the Fund was continuing to take an entirely sound position in including public health and medical economics among its major fields of activity."[53]

However, the opposition of some leaders of the American Medical Association to some of the Fund's activities came to the fore. Some of this may have been due partly to general opposition to any cooperation with the "New Deal" efforts to promote "socialized medicine." Much of it, however, probably was provoked by Kingsbury's speeches rather than by the work of Sydenstricker and Falk. His paper "Adequate Health Service for All the People" presented at the National Conference of Social Work in 1934[54] and his articles of the same year, "Health Insurance for the American People"[55] and "Mutualizing Medical Costs,"[56] probably incited resentment among some medical practitioners of that day.

In January 1935, Albert G. Milbank delivered a paper, "The Relationship of the Milbank Memorial Fund to the Field of Health and the Medical Profession," at the Annual Conference of Secretaries of the County Medical Societies of Indiana, held at Indianapolis. The paper was intended as a peace offering. Mr. Milbank began by summarizing some of the complaints that had been made by medical groups: " . . . the Fund has been charged with advocating State Medicine; of seeking to demote members of the medical profession to the level of government clerks; of placing the emphasis on the quantity of medical care rather than on the quality of medical care; of destroying that priceless human as well as traditional professional relationship between doctor and patient which has been one of the glories of the medical profession from time out of mind; of regimenting and sovietizing a group whose training costs more in time and money than the training of almost any other group in the country and of blaming the doctors because many people do not receive adequate medical care."[57]

He briefly summarized the history of the Fund, described the purposes and results of the three health demonstrations, and stated that the Board of Directors did not question their value.

"As to methods of meeting the costs of medical care, however, a different situation exists. Here the Directors have taken no action, nor, for that matter, has any recommendation on this subject been made to the Directors by the Technical Board. In this matter, the staff of the Fund, with the knowledge and informal approval of the Directors, has conducted a series of studies as to methods in operation in this country and in procedures in operation in many other countries set up to deal with this problem. No final report of these studies has been made. In fact, the studies themselves have not been completed. Interim reports embodying tentative proposals have been released by the staff for the purpose of encouraging discussion and criticism. Therefore the Directors of the Fund are free to take any one of three courses in relation to this subject: (1) They may concur in whole or in part with such conclusions; (2) They may favor some other solution of the problem; or (3) They may abstain from taking any position whatever and simply make the studies of the staff available to those interested in the subject."[58]

Appealing to the statesmanship of the medical profession and extending an offer of closer cooperation, Mr. Milbank continued:

"Our Fund must look in the future to the medical profession for advice more than it has in the past. I urge your profession not to repeat, in this matter of the public aspects of medical costs, what many of your leaders have told me was a mistaken attitude on the part of the profession at the inception of the public health movement . . ."[59]

" . . . the Fund and the various branches of the medical profession, the public health and social welfare workers, the hospital and nursing groups, and the voluntary agencies are all interested and have their place in this broad subject of health. The field is so vast and is capable of such enormous development that there is room and to spare for all of us. There is no need to step on each other's toes. There is every reason for us to go forward in orderly ranks and with irresistible power. No outside force—not even the Government—will seek to withstand our united strength if we are willing to do a good job."[60]

By the spring of 1935, the differences that had developed between the Secretary and several members of the Board and the Technical Board were sufficiently pronounced to make the Secretary's position most uncomfortable—if not untenable. After an exchange of letters between Mr. Kingsbury and Mr. Milbank in which each acknowledged the existence of differences regarding Fund policy, John

Kingsbury's resignation was announced 19 April 1935. As recorded in the previous day's minutes of the Meeting of the Technical Board:

"Mr. Kingsbury then, in adjourning the meeting, bade the members goodnight and goodbye. He said, 'In the words of the late Mr. Justice Holmes to one of the attendants in the Supreme Court, as the venerable Judge was leaving that august body for the last time, I will not be in in the morning.' I declare this meeting adjourned."

In the same fashion, Kingsbury maintained his self-possession during his last day at the office. He called an immediate meeting of the entire staff early in the afternoon of 18 April 1935. Before leaving his desk, this writer had heard a whispered rumor that Kingsbury was to announce his resignation. Quietly Kingsbury stated that he wanted to discuss briefly some of the Fund's work and, in particular, to report on his visit to Yugoslavia. The talk lasted nearly 45 minutes and Kingsbury was especially proud to show the group slides taken on his trip to Yugoslavia, including pictures of the John Kingsbury Health Home at Pranjane and the Elizabeth Milbank Anderson Health Home at Slovak.[61] He then summarized the events of the past few months leading to his resignation and, with tears in his eyes, bade each member of the staff goodbye.

A statement of appreciation for Mr. Kingsbury's past services appeared in the minutes of the 16 May 1935 meeting of the Technical Board and contained such passages as:

The members of the Technical Board of the Milbank Memorial Fund would not let the occasion of its first meeting without Mr. Kingsbury pass, without noting in its Minutes its keen sense of loss due to the absence from the meeting of a remarkable and congenial personality. As originator of the idea of the Technical Board and as its leader, he has done much to give the organization its distinctive qualities.

We would, also, at this time note the unique contribution to public health which Mr. Kingsbury has made during the period of his identification with the Milbank Fund. Through his special genius as an organizer of public opinion he has added significantly to popular understanding of the meaning and possibilities of public health. . . . At times he has been accused by some of wanting to achieve [the] possibilities of preventive health too quickly . . . no one, however, has accused him of lacking earnestness and conviction in his desire to make preventive medicine a great and immediate instrument of improving the positive health and efficiency of all the population, and particularly of that part which does not have adequate access to either preventive or therapeutic medical attention. . . .

In all his efforts he has insisted that public health should be something more than popular. He recognized at all times that it must have the soundest scientific basis. With this in mind, he assembled an extraordinary group of national advisers which, over this period of years, have [sic] influenced the development of public health in this country . . .[62]

### Accession of Edgar Sydenstricker

Edgar Sydenstricker was named Scientific Director of the Milbank Memorial Fund shortly after Kingsbury's resignation. At the 16 May 1935 meeting of the Technical Board, Franklin B. Kirkbride, representing the Board of Directors, announced that Mr. Sydenstricker preferred not to be a member of the Technical Board but would "act as the representative of the Fund's staff and serve as Chairman."

Mr. Sydenstricker let it be known that, as Scientific Director, he would emphasize the research activity of the Fund. This point of view was natural; he had come to the Fund nine years earlier to study the statistical aspects of the health demonstrations and, since 1928, had been Chief of the Division of Research (which he had founded). Current research studies included maternity and infancy studies by Dorothy G. Wiehl; studies in tuberculosis by Jean Downes; the continuing health insurance studies of Dr. Falk; studies in population by Drs. Notestein and Kiser; the new studies of family planning in Spartanburg, South Carolina, and Cincinnati, Ohio, by Dr. Regine K. Stix under Dr. Notestein's direction; the school health education project in Cattaraugus of Ruth Grout; and the public health nursing studies of Marian G. Randall.

At the 14 November 1935 meeting of the Technical Board, Mr. Sydenstricker announced that within a month Dr. Falk would complete the studies in the field of medical care that had been authorized under the formal program of the Fund. He requested advice as to whether the Fund should definitely conclude or continue its work in this field. If the work was to continue, should the Fund itself perform these studies or simply assist other agencies to perform them? Opinion on these matters was divided. Three medical members of the Technical Board felt that further studies should be conducted under medical auspices *assisted* by the Fund. "Dr. Falk observed that the subject was so controversial that it would lead to difficulties no matter how it was undertaken, that if the Fund were to sponsor further studies [in medical care] it should do so only out of basic conviction, and that if, on the other hand, the Fund should assist other organizations—lay or medical—a definite agreement should be reached absolving the Fund from responsibility."[63]

The Board of Directors apparently heeded Dr. Falk's advice. At all events, there was a temporary suspension of Fund activity in medical care. Dr. Falk's own book, *Security Against Sickness,* appeared in 1936,[64] and he himself left the Fund in that year. With the exception of occasional papers on medical care prepared by others for the *Quarterly* or for the Annual Conference, the Fund ceased for some time direct activity in the field of medical care.

Sydenstricker, however, had sufficient work to busy both himself and the staff. He was thoroughly involved with the problems of the National Health Survey; in January 1936, he induced the present writer to go to Detroit for six months, initially to help in administering the occupational mortality and morbidity unit and later to plan tabulations of the fertility data being collected by the Survey, which were to be assigned to the Fund for analysis. During Sydenstricker's early months as Scientific Director, he had frequent talks with Harold W. Dodds, Frederick Osborn, Albert G. Milbank, Frank W. Notestein, and others concerning the Fund's possible assistance in establishing an Office of Population Research within the Woodrow Wilson School of Public and International Affairs at Princeton University. In accordance with this plan, Frank W. Notestein would be appointed Director of the Office.

Although a good administrator, who apparently enjoyed his role as Scientific Director, Sydenstricker seemed to find unduly time-consuming his new duties: reading appeals, meeting an endless stream of visitors, and arranging meetings of the Board and Technical Board.

After discussing the matter, Mr. Milbank and Mr. Sydenstricker agreed that the solution might be to find an able administrative assistant who could "front" for Sydenstricker and so afford him more time to devote to policy and general future programs. It was decided that since Sydenstricker was not a medical person the assistant should have this qualification. Dr. Frank G. Boudreau, who had been Sydenstricker's successor at the Health Office of the League of Nations, seemed to have the proper qualifications. Furthermore, Dr. Boudreau had written to Mr. Sydenstricker and indicated an interest in seeking a different position. In a letter dated 10 March 1936, Edgar Sydenstricker outlined his needs to Dr. Boudreau and asked if he would allow his name to be considered by the Board for the position of Sydenstricker's "associate, possibly with some such title as 'Medical Director'."

At the beginning of 1936, the Scientific Director appeared to have other office matters well under control. Drs. Lowell J. Reed and Wade H. Frost of Johns Hopkins University were elected as members of the Technical Board in January, 1936. At the 20 February 1936 meeting of the Technical Board, Mr. Sydenstricker outlined, in some detail, plans for the Fourteenth Annual Advisory Conference to be held in March.

On 19 March 1936, a few days before the Conference, while working at his desk in the Fund's offices at 40 Wall Street, Edgar Sydenstricker had a stroke and died a few hours later. He was 56. On his desk were found the final papers, recently signed, concerning the plans to establish the Office of Population Research at Princeton University.

Because John A. Kingsbury and Edgar Sydenstricker operated as a team during 1926–1935, they have been considered in the same chapter. During 1922–1935, Kingsbury served as head under the title of Secretary. He served without Sydenstricker's help for the first four years only. For two years (1926–1927), Sydenstricker served with Kingsbury as a consultant and for seven years (1928–1935) as Director of the Division of Research; he held the position of Scientific Director for scarcely a year.

Kingsbury's major achievement was the basic organization of the

New York Health Demonstrations, together with the idea of creating a technical board and an advisory council to plan and guide the demonstrations. The *Milbank Memorial Fund Quarterly Bulletin* and the Annual Conferences of the Advisory Council were also initiated early in Kingsbury's tenure.

Sydenstricker's outstanding contributions included the introduction of stricter statistical monitoring of the health demonstrations, the establishment of a Division of Research to study selected problems of public health, the initiation of research in population and family planning as topics of relevance to health, and the transformation of the *Milbank Memorial Fund Quarterly Bulletin* from a small house organ to a scientific journal of public health and demography. Sydenstricker was able to make those contributions because he had the confidence and the backing of the Secretary, the Technical Board, and the Board of Directors.

Kingsbury and Sydenstricker shared a deep interest in and concern with problems of health and social welfare. In addition to support of the New York Health Demonstrations and the Committee on the Costs of Medical Care, important grants which further reflect the interests of either Kingsbury or Sydenstricker were those to the East Harlem Health Center and the New York Tuberculosis and Health Association, those which provided for the founding and initial support of the International Union for the Scientific Study of Population, and those to Princeton University, which included establishment of the Office of Population Research.

## References

[1] Minutes of the 11 May 1921 meeting of the Board, at which the action of the Special Committee was approved.

[2] *Milbank Memorial Fund, Report for the Year Ended December 31, 1922 with Historical Summary* (New York: Milbank Memorial Fund, 1923), p. 16.

[3] As stated by Winslow, "The Commonwealth Fund Demonstrations were begun later —at Fargo, North Dakota, in 1923; in Clarke County, Georgia, and Rutherford County, Tennessee, in 1924, and in Marion County, Oregon, in 1925." C.-E. A. Winslow, *Health on the Farm and in the Village* (New York: The Macmillan Company, 1931), p. 38.

[4] *Milbank Memorial Fund, Report for the Year Ended December 21, 1922 . . .* , p. 16.

[5] Appendix 5 provides a complete list of past and current members of the Technical Board.

[6] Minutes, Meeting of the Board of Directors, 22 May 1922.

[7] C.-E. A. Winslow, *Health on the Farm and in the Village* (New York: The Macmillan Company, 1931).

C.-E. A. Winslow, *A City Set on a Hill* (Garden City, N.Y.: Doubleday, Doran & Company, 1934).

C.-E. A. Winslow and Savel Zimand, *Health Under the "El"* (New York: Harper & Brothers, 1937).

[8] Winslow, *Health on the Farm and in the Village,* p. 43.

[9] According to Smillie, "Jefferson County, Kentucky (1908) and Guilford County, North Carolina (1911); each claim priority in the establishment of full time county health unit service." See Wilson G. Smillie, *Public Health Administration in the United States* (New York: The Macmillan Company, 1935), p. 315.

[10] Winslow, *Health on the Farm and in the Village,* p. 1.

[11] *Ibid.,* pp. 44–45.

[12] *Ibid.,* p. 142.

[13] *Ibid.,* p. 242.

[14] *Ibid.,* p. 243.

[15] *Ibid.,* pp. 208, 221–223.

[16] Winslow, *A City Set on a Hill,* p. 61.

[17] *Ibid.,* p. 62.

[18] *Ibid.,* pp. 73–75.

[19] *Ibid.,* p. 73.

[20] C.-E. A. Winslow and Savel Zimand, *Health Under the "El"* (New York and London: Harper & Brothers, 1937), p. 44.

[21] *Ibid.,* pp. 44–45.

[22] *Ibid.,* p. 52.

[23] *Ibid.,* pp. 91–92. In a footnote about this situation, the authors state, "In the spring of 1929, interviews were had by a representative of the demonstration with 104 physicians in the district who were known to have more or less practice in the field of venereal disease, in an attempt to find out whether there was a need for such diagnostic facilities as had been provided, and might be reopened, and whether they could profitably use nursing service supplied through the demonstration in following up their cases. No enthusiasm for either proposal was uncovered by these interviews." *Ibid.,* p. 92.

[24] *Ibid.,* p. 96.

[25] *Ibid.,* pp. 185–186.

[26] Harry L. Hopkins, "Health Planning in the Recovery Program," *Problems of*

*Health Conservation,* Proceedings of the Twelfth Annual Conference of the Milbank Memorial Fund, held March 14–15, 1934, at the New York Academy of Medicine (New York: Milbank Memorial Fund, 1934), pp. 84–91. Hopkins became a protege of Kingsbury in 1912, while the latter was with A.I.C.P. Rejected for army service, Hopkins left A.I.C.P. in 1917 to serve with the Red Cross. He rejoined A.I.C.P. in 1921, with the assistance of Kingsbury, who was then engaged in work for the Milbank Memorial Fund. See Robert E. Sherwood, *Roosevelt and Hopkins* (New York: Harper and Brothers, 1948), pp. 23 and 27. While with A.I.C.P., Hopkins helped with some preliminary surveys of the Bellevue-Yorkville area in preparation for the demonstration (Winslow and Zimand, *op. cit.,* p. 40).

[27] Winslow and Zimand, *op. cit.,* p. x.

[28] "The demonstrations were initiated in 1922, when 8.4 per cent of the Fund's total disbursements of that year were devoted to them. The peak year of expenditures on the demonstrations was 1925 when 57 per cent of the Fund's total financial outlay was for these projects. The percentage of the Fund's annual gifts devoted to the demonstrations has gradually declined since that date. In 1929, the demonstration expenditures were 34.3 per cent of the total. Marked reductions in the Fund's financial participation in the Cattaraugus County and Syracuse health demonstrations are largely responsible for the decrease, because payments toward the Bellevue-Yorkville Health Demonstration, the last organized, have increased annually since 1925, the peak year to date having been in 1929." *Milbank Memorial Fund, Annual Report for 1929* (New York: Milbank Memorial Fund, 1930), pp. 17–18.

[29] The first appointee (1915) as a statistician in the United States Public Health Service, Sydenstricker had supervised the statistical work of the Service in studies of pellagra, influenza, and industrial hygiene. In 1923, he went to Geneva on leave "to act as Chief of Service of Epidemiological Intelligence and Public Health Statistics for the League of Nations in initiating the statistical work of the League's health organization" *Milbank Memorial Fund Quarterly Bulletin* 3 (January 1926): 12.

[30] Edgar Sydenstricker, "The Measurement of Results of Public Health Work: An Introductory Discussion," *1926 Annual Report of the Milbank Memorial Fund* (New York: Milbank Memorial Fund, 1927), p. 35.

[31] Edgar Sydenstricker, "The Statistical Evaluation of the Results of Social Experiments in Public Health," *Proceedings of the American Statistical Association,* Proceedings Supplement 161A (1928): 165.

[32] Dorothy G. Wiehl, "Infant Mortality in Cattaraugus County," *The Milbank Memorial Fund Quarterly Bulletin* 6 (January 1928): 23.

[33] Dorothy G. Wiehl, "The Correction of Infant Mortality Rates for Residence," *American Journal of Public Health* Vol. 19, No. 5 (May 1929): 495–510. Jean Downes, "The Accuracy of the Recorded Birth Statistics in Urban and Rural Areas," *Journal of the American Statistical Association* 24 (March 1929): 15–27.

[34] See C. V. Kiser, "The Work of the Milbank Memorial Fund in Population Since 1928," *Forty Years of Research in Human Fertility: Retrospect and Prospect, The Milbank Memorial Fund Quarterly* 49 (Part 2, October 1971): 5–62.

[35] In 1923, when the *Milbank Memorial Fund Quarterly Bulletin* was started as a

means of disseminating information about the health demonstrations, Bertrand Brown joined the staff of the Milbank Memorial Fund as editorial assistant. He was named Assistant Secretary of the Fund in 1925 and Director of the newly created Division of Publications in 1929; he retired from the Fund 31 December 1933. Edgar Sydenstricker became Editor with the January 1934 issue, which was the first to delete the word "Bulletin" from the masthead. See *Milbank Memorial Fund Quarterly* 12 (January 1934): 2.

[36] The need for additional office space was an important reason for moving from the original headquarters at 49 Wall Street to the newly erected Bank of Manhattan Building, 40 Wall Street, in the spring of 1932. This has continued as the Fund's address to the present day.

[37] The 1936 *Annual Report* of the Fund contained the following statement:

> It is with deep regret that I record the death, on October 29, 1936, of Thomas Cochran, a member of the Fund's Board of Directors since 1921. Mr. Cochran became a member of the Board upon the direct invitation of Elizabeth Milbank Anderson, founder of the Fund, at a time when Mrs. Anderson, with a full realization that she had but a short time to live, turned her thoughts to the future of the Fund and to the steps she might take to insure its continued usefulness.
>
> While in accord with the Fund's efforts to establish better standards of health, Mr. Cochran expressed, on occasion, his concern about some of the social and economic implications which are inherent in a longer life expectancy. He therefore urged at an early date a study of population problems and interrelated subjects. As a direct result of Mr. Cochran's interest in this subject, the Fund embarked on certain preliminary studies within this particular field of inquiry. These population studies have been followed by an ever-increasing emphasis upon this important subject, with the result that contributions of marked significance have been made by the Fund in a field which affects the economic, social, and political life of the nations of the world.

Quoted from *Milbank Memorial Fund, Annual Report for 1936* (New York: Milbank Memorial Fund, 1937), pp. iv–v. See also *Forty Years of Research in Human Fertility: Retrospect and Prospect, The Milbank Memorial Fund Quarterly* 49 (Part 2, October 1971): 20, 69.

[38] Ray Lyman Wilbur, "Foreword," *The Five Year Program of the Committee on the Costs of Medical Care,* Publication No. 1 of the Committee on the Costs of Medical Care (Washington, D.C., 1928), p. 6.

[39] Elizabeth Fox was subsequently succeeded by John Sundwall.

[40] Wilbur, *op. cit.,* p. 7.

[41] A. G. Milbank, "Socialized Capitalism," *Survey Graphic* (July 1932).

[42] *Medical Care for the American People: The Final Report of the Committee on the Costs of Medical Care* (Chicago: University of Chicago Press, 1932). Recommendation 1 appears on p. 109; recommendation 2, on p. 118; recommendation 3, on p. 120; recommendation 4 on pp. 134–135; and recommendation 5, on p. 138.

[43] *Milbank Memorial Fund, Annual Report for 1932* (New York: Milbank Memorial Fund, 1933), p. 21.

[44] *Milbank Memorial Fund, Annual Report for 1933* (New York: Milbank Memorial Fund, 1934), pp. 20–21.

[45] Minutes, Technical Board Meeting, 16 February 1933.

[46] Minutes, Technical Board Meeting, 15 June 1933.

[47] Early in 1933, Sydenstricker took advantage of an opportunity to utilize the help of white-collar workers from the "Emergency Work Bureau" of New York City to collect data on health and fertility in relation to economic conditions. This work was done in the Bushwick section of Brooklyn and in Harlem. Later that year, the Fund was invited by the U.S.P.H.S. to assist in collecting somewhat similar data in selected poor areas of ten cities. This, in turn, served as a "proving ground" for the organization of the National Health Survey of 1935–36, conducted by the U.S.P.H.S. with funds from the Works Progress Administration. The Fund's participation in the National Health Survey will be described later.

The "Health and Depression" studies conducted by the Fund and U.S.P.H.S. under Sydenstricker's leadership during the early thirties supplemented those made by the Committee on the Costs of Medical Care and underlined the close relationship of unemployment and diminishing income to amount of sickness and inadequacy of medical care.

[48] Sir Arthur Newsholme and John Adams Kingsbury, *Red Medicine: Socialized Health in Soviet Russia* (Garden City, New York: Doubleday, Doran & Company, 1933). It should be noted that this book was not a publication of the Milbank Memorial Fund and carried no explicit imprimatur from the Fund. However, on the title page Kingsbury's title is listed as "Secretary of the Milbank Memorial Fund, Formerly Commissioner of Public Charities, City of New York." In the introduction, after stating the reasons for their exploratory study of health conditions in the U.S.S.R., the authors state on page 2, ". . . a joint visit of inquiry was then initiated on behalf of the Milbank Memorial Fund." Also, in the Preface the authors "appreciate deeply the generous aid of the Milbank Memorial Fund in enabling us to pursue this study." Page ix, furthermore, carries the statement that they "are indebted to Victor O. Freeburg, of the staff of the Milbank Memorial Fund, for editorial assistance and for seeing the book through the press."

[49] Minutes, Technical Board Meeting, 2 February 1933.

[50] Minutes, Technical Board Meeting, 18 January 1934.

[51] Minutes, Technical Board Meeting, 14 June 1934.

[52] Minutes, Technical Board Meeting, 18 October 1934.

[53] Minutes, Technical Board Meetings, 6 December 1934.

[54] *Adequate Health for All*, proceedings of the National Conference of Social Work (Chicago: University of Chicago Press, 1934) pp. 304–324.

[55] *Western Hospital Review* No. 3 (May 1934): 5, 17–19.

[56] *Survey Graphic*, xxiii, No. 6 (June 1934): 285–286, 295.

[57] A. G. Milbank, "The Relationship of the Milbank Memorial Fund to the Field of Health and the Medical Profession," *The Milbank Memorial Fund Quarterly* 13 (April 1935): 100.

[58] *Ibid.*, p. 102.

[59] *Ibid.*, p. 111.

[60] *Ibid.*, p. 120.

[61] Kingsbury was justly proud of his role in the development of health centers in Yugoslavia following the ravages suffered by that country in World War I. As Chairman of the Executive Committee of the Serbian Relief Committee, he had visited Yugoslavia in 1920 and was doubtless instrumental in persuading the Memorial Fund Association to make a grant to the Serbian Relief Committee during that same year. In an article, "Yugoslavia Leads in Rural Health Centers," published in 1934, Freeburg stated, "The establishment of these health centers, one after another during the last twelve years, is a heroic achievement of reconstruction, which has already provided old Serbian Yugoslavia with a more extensive health organization of the rural masses than can be found in any similar area, except perhaps in Denmark. . . . How effectively the Yugoslavians had been able to organize their own resources was observed in 1932, during a tour of inspection, by John A. Kingsbury, secretary of the Milbank Memorial Fund, chairman of the executive committee of the Serbian Child Welfare Association in America, who attended the dedication of the King Alexander I Health Home. Mr. Kingsbury, as he went from center to center, was deeply impressed by the change from the terrible conditions which he had witnessed in 1920. . . ."

Victor O. Freeburg, "Yugoslavia Leads in Rural Health Centers," *The Milbank Memorial Fund Quarterly* 12 (January 1934): 15. This article contains a picture, on page 17, of the John Kingsbury Health Home. An illustration of the Elizabeth Milbank Anderson Health Home appears on page 10 of *Thirty-Five Years in Review* (New York: Milbank Memorial Fund, 1940).

[62] Minutes, Technical Board Meeting, 16 May 1934.

[63] Minutes, Technical Board Meeting, 14 November 1935.

[64] I. S. Falk, *Security Against Sickness* (Garden City, New York: Doubleday, Doran & Co., 1936).

# Chapter 4

# Twenty-five Years with
# Frank G. Boudreau, 1937–1962

SHORTLY BEFORE HIS DEATH Edgar Sydenstricker had written to Dr. Frank G. Boudreau, to ask whether he would be interested in joining the Milbank Memorial Fund as the Scientific Director's administrative assistant. However, Sydenstricker's sudden death created an immediate need for an Executive Director. After talking with other members of the Board of Directors, Albert G. Milbank himself entered into correspondence with Dr. Boudreau.

After several exchanges of letters, a strong feeling of mutual respect had developed—and the possibility of Dr. Boudreau's appointment as Executive Director. It was arranged that Dr. Boudreau would visit the Fund after he had completed an American assignment for the League of Nations during the fall of 1936. Upon his arrival he was given a desk in the Fund's offices and invited to attend the 15 October and the 17 December 1936 meetings of the Technical Board. At the October meeting he described some of the activities of the Health Secretariat of the League of Nations. At the December meeting he was requested to "comment upon the significance of the trip which he had arranged for Latin American professors of hygiene in America," which had been his mission for the League. Shortly thereafter, at the December meeting of the Board of Directors, Dr. Boudreau briefly described his principal interests and presented his ideas about promising lines of research for a foundation in the field of health. Boudreau later thanked Milbank for his skillful and sympathetic handling of a meeting which might have been trying but proved most enjoyable.

71

Dr. Boudreau, born of American parents in Canada 18 July 1886, had taken the M.D. degree at McGill in 1910. He had been serving as Chief of the Communicable Disease Section of the Ohio State Department of Health when he was appointed to the Health Section of the League of Nations in 1925.

The appointment of Dr. Boudreau as Executive Director of the Milbank Memorial Fund was decided upon shortly after his talk with the members of the Board. Before returning to Geneva, he held a meeting of those on the Milbank staff who were responsible for planning the Annual Conference in the spring of 1937. He returned to New York for full-time service with the Fund on 1 April 1937.

Dr. Boudreau viewed the Conference of 1937 as a fortunate opportunity to observe, at first hand, results of some of the Fund's current work and the experts' reception of the research reports. It gave him the chance to meet and become better acquainted with a large group of leaders in public health and demography, and he himself won praise for his success in securing John Winant, of the International Labor Office, as principal speaker at the Annual Dinner.[1]

Soon after he began his duties as Executive Director of the Milbank Memorial Fund, Dr. Boudreau let it be known that he intended to explore the field of nutrition as a possible new area for research. For this purpose, he employed Dr. Harry D. Kruse, a biological chemist at Johns Hopkins University and editor of the *American Journal of Hygiene*. Reporting for work in the fall of 1937, Dr. Kruse's first assignment was to review the literature on current work in nutrition and to visit various universities and centers performing notable research in that field.

Dr. Boudreau introduced another new area of interest to the Fund: the public health aspects of housing. This was, however, largely confined to support of the work of Dr. C.-E.A. Winslow, as Chairman of the American Public Health Association's Committee on the Public Health Aspects of Housing, which was sponsored by the Health Organization of the League of Nations.

To make room for these new fields of research, there was a gradual and orderly termination of several existing projects. A few months after his arrival, Dr. Boudreau expressed a wish to discontinue the

Fund's studies of contraception after existing commitments were completed.[2]

Further curtailment of the Fund's previous areas of research was achieved simply by failing to replace several staff members who left the Fund for other positions. Thus the Fund's research in community nursing terminated when Marian Randall left in 1937. No effort was made to replace Dr. Ralph E. Wheeler on his departure in 1939.

Dr. Boudreau soon manifested a desire to continue some population research at the Fund in addition to the Fund's support to the Office of Population Research at Princeton. He quickly affirmed that the Fund would keep its commitment to analyze and prepare a report on the fertility data that were collected by the National Health Survey of 1935–36. In 1939, the Fund accepted a grant from the Carnegie Corporation of New York to enable it to sponsor a cooperative study of social and psychological factors affecting fertility; P. K. Whelpton of the Scripps Foundation for Research in Population Problems was field director of this study. He and the present writer edited the series of reports in the Indianapolis study.[3]

Dr. Kruse's exploratory survey of research in nutrition involved visits to the outstanding centers of research in the field. His report, "Results of Recent Research in Nutrition," published in 1940 in the *Proceedings of the Conference on Convalescent Care,* held at the New York Academy of Medicine in 1939, not only gave the broad findings of his investigations but served to define the aspects of nutrition with which the Fund was to be concerned:

> By their very nature, nutrition and diet are closely associated. Despite the intimate relationship between them, their fundamentally different meanings and their separate spheres make it desirable to restore the original distinction between them. Nutrition as a term, . . . is a bodily process. Diet, on the contrary, comprises the foodstuffs which are consumed for use in the body. It supports the bodily process. . . .[4]
>
> According to present criteria of adequacy in diets, the amount of protein and number of calories, which have served so long as bases of judgment, are still decisive

points; but now others must also be included. For one
thing, there is the biological value of the protein, depend-
ing in part on the presence of at least eleven indispensable
amino acids. Then too, sixteen other chemical substances
are known to be essential in the diet: vitamin A, vitamin
B1 (thiamin), vitamin G (riboflavin), factor P-P (nicotin-
ic acid), vitamin C (ascorbic acid), vitamin D, linoleic or
linolenic acid, calcium, phosphorus, magnesium, sodium,
potassium, chlorine, iodine, iron, and manganese. And the
list is not yet complete.[5]

Much of Kruse's research at the Fund concerned ocular manifes-
tations of ariboflavinosis and other nutritional deficiencies.

Dr. Boudreau early expressed interest in continuing the research
being carried out by Dorothy G. Wiehl and Jean Downes, both of
whom had begun to focus their work upon the area of nutrition. In
fact, as described later, Dorothy Wiehl took a leading role in three extensive inductive studies which directly concerned nutrition or bore
closely upon it.

In 1940 a cooperative study on the medical evaluation of nutri-
tional status was begun under the auspices of the Departments of
Public Health and Preventive Medicine and of Pediatrics of Cornell
University Medical College, the Milbank Memorial Fund, the New
York City Department of Health, and the Division of Public Health
Methods of the United States Public Health Service. Representatives
of these organizations constituted the General Committee for the
Study: Frank G. Boudreau, H.D. Kruse, Samuel Z. Levine, Carroll E.
Palmer, George T. Palmer, Thomas Parran, George St. J. Perrott,
William Schmidt, Wilson G. Smillie, and Dorothy G. Wiehl. Dorothy
Wiehl was chiefly responsible for the conduct of the study, whose
principal research area was nutrition among children in two schools:
one in a poor area of the Lower East Side and one in a well-to-do
suburban area.

Since it was funded by the Works Progress Administration, the
study bore a resemblance to the National Health Survey of 1935–36.
In addition to the scientific goals, an important reason for the investigation was the creation of jobs for unemployed white-collar workers.

Although the nutrition study was born of the depression, the outbreak of European war in 1939 increased interest in nutrition and emphasized the need for more research in the field. With his Canadian background, Boudreau quite naturally became interested in that country's work in nutrition. Dr. Frederick F. Tisdall, Wing Commander of the Canadian Royal Air Force, became a frequent visitor at the Fund and a virtual co-worker with Dr. Kruse. He and several Canadian colleagues, all in uniform, were frequently at Technical Board meetings during the early forties, reporting on progress made in fortifying foods with the essential vitamins.

In 1941, a Food and Nutrition Board, with Dr. Boudreau as Chairman, was organized within the National Research Council. Among the members were H. D. Kruse, F. F. Tisdall, and Glen King who had earlier isolated vitamin C and later became a member of the Fund's Board of Directors and Technical Board. To provide data needed by the Food and Nutrition Board, the Fund launched a statistical study examining the relationship of vitamins and nutritional status to the work performance of aircraft workers. Again, Dorothy Wiehl had a key role.

The last large study of nutrition conducted by the Fund concerned the relationship between nutrition of pregnant women and the outcome of pregnancy and health of the infant and mother. The "Maternal and Newborn Nutrition Studies at Philadelphia Lying-In Hospital" were cooperatively supported by the Milbank Memorial Fund, the Williams-Waterman Fund, the National Vitamin Foundation, the Upjohn Company, E. R. Squibb and Sons, and, in part, by the Nutrition Foundation and Mead Johnson & Company. There were six reports of findings, most of them prepared by Richard V. Kasius and Dorothy G. Wiehl of the Fund's staff; Winslow T. Tompkins, formerly Director of Nutrition Studies at Pennsylvania Hospital; and Alexander Randall, formerly Pediatric Fellow, Nutrition Studies, Pennsylvania Hospital.

Jean Downes's research, during Dr. Boudreau's regime, was also frequently related to nutrition. It included a study of the correlation between nutrition and tuberculosis among Harlem Negroes. Her main activity during 1938–43, however, was the supervision of a study of illness among a sample of families in the Eastern Health District of Baltimore, Maryland. This was a cooperative effort, which involved the Fund, the Public Health Service, Baltimore City Health Department, and Johns Hopkins University. Under the general title, "Family Studies in the Eastern Health District," the series of reports was published in the *Quarterly* over a period of years.

In addition to the Indianapolis study, the Fund's population studies under Dr. Boudreau's directorship included preparation of the volume, *Group Differences in Urban Fertility,* based upon data from The National Health Survey; cooperation with the Bureau of the Census, and the Social Science Research Council in getting out the 1950 Census Monograph *The Fertility of American Women*; cooperation with the American Public Health Association's Committee on Vital and Health Statistics relating to the 1960 Census period; and continued support of the Office of Population Research and its Princeton Fertility Survey. The postwar round tables on population, held in connection with the Fund's Annual Conferences, focused on demographic aspects of modernization.[6]

Dr. Boudreau's continued interest in nutrition and health was crowned by the important roles that he played in the establishment of the Food and Agriculture Organization of the United Nations and of the World Health Organization. He took part in drafting the constitution and bylaws of both and in selecting their original leaders, Lord Boyd Orr, the first Director of the F.A.O., and Dr. Brock Chisholm, the first Director-General of W.H.O. He also encouraged the organization of the Citizens Committee for W.H.O. in this country.

Early in 1948, Dr. Boudreau announced that several meetings of the Technical Board would focus their attention on the subject of mental hygiene, including the teaching of mental health in schools of public health. This was the first sign of a possibility that the Fund might shift its attention to mental health, as its interest in nutrition was declining, following the successful accomplishment of several goals in that area.

Historical precedence for the Fund's entrance into the field of mental health could be furnished by Mrs. Elizabeth Milbank Anderson's concern with the problem. She had befriended Clifford W. Beers, author of *A Mind that Found Itself.* Moreover, during the second decade of the century, the Memorial Fund Association had made several grants to the National Committee on Mental Hygiene.

The subsequent developments came shortly after the passage of the 1947 National Mental Health Act which heralded the first major effort in the mental health field by the federal government. The Charter of the World Health Organization, in the drafting of which Dr. Boudreau played a significant leadership role, had also included in its definition of health the phrase "physical, mental and social well-being. . ." which laid the foundation for many governments to include mental health in their main health programs. Perhaps he felt that the Fund had made all the contribution it could in nutrition, and that these new signs of changed government initiatives afforded an opportunity for the Fund to provide leadership in a newly developing aspect of public health work. In implementing this idea, Dr. Boudreau brought together several other earlier experiences.

Believing that epidemiology forms the scientific foundation for all disease control programs, he took the initiative in bringing together leading epidemiologists and leading psychiatrists to explore the potential of developing an epidemiology of mental disorder. The monograph which emerged from that meeting, *Epidemiology of Mental Disorder* (1949), was the Fund's first monograph in the mental health field and the first monograph ever published on this topic.

Dr. Ernest M. Gruenberg, who was then associated with Yale University's Departments of Psychiatry and Public Health, and Dr. Alexander Leighton, at that time a member of Cornell University's Department of Sociology and Anthropology, participated in the round table. Dr. Leighton presented a proposal for research in the epidemiology of mental disorder, which later developed into his Stirling County Study, initially supported by the Fund.

Having seen the consequences of the local health demonstrations in three New York State communities, Dr. Boudreau paid close attention to the developments of the New York State mental health programs. Franklin B. Kirkbride was still alive at that time, a member of the Fund's Board and a frequent participant in Technical Board meetings. His father, Dr. Thomas Kirkbride, had been one of the thirteen founders of the American Psychiatric Association in 1844 and had designed the first modern mental hospital, which was copied all over the Western world and became known as the Kirkbride Mental Hospital design. Mr. Kirkbride himself was Chairman of the Board of Visitors of Letchworth Village, a state school for the mentally retarded, and had a strong interest in New York State's mental health programs.

The Technical Board included Surgeon General Thomas Parran, formerly New York State Health Commissioner, and his current successor, Dr. Herman Hilleboe. The State legislature had created a temporary Mental Health Commission, part of whose charge was the "development and correlation of mental health activities of public and private agencies operating at the local community level . . . ." Dr. Boudreau took a lively interest in the problem of staffing this Commission and encouraged Dr. Gruenberg to accept the proposal that he become its executive director. He incorporated Dr. Gruenberg and other members of the Commission staff into several Technical Board meetings, and had Dr. Gruenberg's help in organizing several round table meetings at the Fund's Annual Conferences during the subsequent years while the Commission was carrying out its charge. The Commission prepared the 1954 New York State Community Mental Health Services Act, which undid a century's tradition of regarding the mentally ill as "wards of the state." It returned to local government the authority to conduct mental health programs in a new department of local government, which received automatic 50-percent State reimbursement for State-approved programs. This legislation was quickly copied by many of the other major states, and the resulting spate of local community mental health programs throughout the nation laid the groundwork for the National Mental Health Center legislation of 1963.

In 1955, Dr. Boudreau invited Dr. Gruenberg to join the Fund's staff in order to direct its work in mental health. In 1951, Dr. H.D. Kruse had assumed responsibility for a symposium on the biology of mental health and disease. A round table on interrelations between the social environment and psychiatric disorders, at the 1952 Annual Conference, included reports of several current research projects, among them the Stirling County study and those of the New York State Mental Health Research Unit under the direction of Dr. Gruenberg, Executive Director of the Mental Health Commission.

The 1955 Annual Conference saw the convening of a round table on the elements of a community mental health program. At this Conference also, Samuel R. Milbank, who had been President of the Fund since 1952,[7] "announced the Fund's intention to seek ways and means of implementing demonstration community mental health programs, together with intensive quantitative evaluations, so that the opportunities now emerging for increased size and strength of community mental health programs would have the greatest possible opportunity of being used in constructive and tested activities."[8]

At the 1956 Annual Conference round table on programs for community mental health, Dr. Boudreau announced the appointment of an Advisory Council on Mental Health Demonstrations, to consist of 32 members. In addition, an eight-member Committee on Evaluation had been named.[9] With this action, Dr. Boudreau borrowed from the early days of the health demonstrations a touchstone of their unquestioned success. It will be recalled that an Advisory Council and a Statistical Subcommittee were appointed before the demonstrations began, the Council to review annually or periodically the conduct, progress, and findings of the demonstrations, the Subcommittee to help secure the statistics needed for the selection of survey areas and assist with the preparation of survey instruments.

The 1958 Annual Conference saw a round table on progress and problems of community mental health services present reports on eight mental health services. Six of these related to county services in mental health: San Mateo, California; St. Louis County, Missouri; Minnehaha County, South Dakota; and Monroe, Nassau, and Schnectady Counties, New York. In addition, the mental health services in Quincy, Massachusetts, and the province of Saskatchewan, Canada, were described. The 1958 round table on progress and problems of community mental health services provided an opportunity for the exchange of the rapidly expanding experiences which emerged following the 1954 Community Mental Health Services legislation. Publication of the Conference report shows that problems loomed somewhat larger than progress at that time.

While the community mental health services were developing growing strength, the mental hospitals were showing no sign of fundamental change. The new community services tended to concentrate on a different set of mental health problems, and their growth was not associated with lowered hospital utilization rates. Through the contacts with the World Health Organization another type of community service had come to the Fund's attention in 1953, when Dr. T.P. Rees of England described his program for community care of severely ill mental patients following very brief periods of hospitalization. Dr. Robert C. Hunt, a former New York State mental hospital director who was then assistant commissioner in charge of implementing local community services programs, had met Dr. Rees when he visited New York and was eager to see these programs in action. On the principle that foundations should not undermine the proper functions of government agencies, considerable energy went into persuading the Surgeon General's office to request a traveling fellowship from the World Health Organization for Dr. Hunt to visit Dr. Rees' hospital, Dr. Duncan Macmillan's hospital in Nottingham, England, and Dr. Bell's hospital in Scotland. Dr. Hunt reported that these programs had developed a pattern of community care outside the hospital for the severely ill. He said that the most severe handicaps were much less common when patients were cared for in this way. In 1957, this theme was taken up again in a set of activities which Dr. Boudreau referred to informally as the "Mission to Britain." When Dr. T. P. Rees retired from the directorship of Warlingham Park Hospital, he was engaged by the Fund to conduct a tour of the community care programs in Britain for a committee of New York State Mental Hospital Directors appointed by the Commissioner, Paul Hoch. Their reports on how these programs succeeded in opening the mental hospital doors and running unlocked hospital services for patients who spent most of their time in treatment while at home, coming to the hospital as needed, were supplemented, at the Fund's Annual Conference in 1959, by the reports of similar hospital director committees from Connecticut and New Jersey.

These reports afforded a preview of the seminal impact of those visits on mental hospital administration in the United States. Committee members from New York State included Nathan Beckenstein of the Brooklyn State Hospital, Robert C. Hunt, later of the Hudson River State Hospital, Francis J. O'Neill of the Central Islip State Hospital, Hyman Pleasure of Middletown State Homeopathic Hospital, and Herman B. Snow of St. Lawrence State Hospital.

Dr. Snow was the first to apply fully the lessons learned in England by unlocking all the doors of the St. Lawrence State Hospital.

However, it was Dr. Francis J. O'Neill who helped to promote national awareness of the possibilities:

> I was one of the skeptics who went to Britain, and I was not convinced from what I saw in Britain that I could apply it to my very large hospital. I well remember the last conference we hospital directors had together in London just before we scattered to the four winds in January of 1957.
>
> At that time I said that I did not believe that I would be able to extend the open ward program to Central Islip to any great extent.
>
> When I came back, I was scared. The implications of this program were so startling to me that I was really frightened for my position, for my hospital, and for everyone involved in it. Nevertheless, we went ahead orienting our employees and our patients and orienting our community.
>
> Since the community that surrounds my hospital is made up largely of employees of my hospital, indoctrinating the employees to this program, meant that we were also indoctrinating the community. I also felt that community attitudes and acceptance would be very good because of this fact.
>
> I remember one of my first statements to my staff when I got back was that I would aim for a 30 per cent open ward program in two years. Yet after two years this very large public mental hospital now has 7,172 patients living on open wards; that is 71.5 per cent of the patients. An additional 604 patients, or another six per cent have ground privileges which is equivalent to open word privileges excepting that these patients come from closed wards.
>
> Our program has developed as a fairly permissive one. The patient who is on an open ward has almost unlimited freedom of the grounds. There are very few exceptions to this.
>
> Several things have happened to us since this program started. We went along very well for about a year with good community acceptance, with a gradual development of an open program, and acceptance by our employees way

beyond what I had expected, when last September I returned from my vacation to find the community up in
arms. A few residents who had come to the area from other regions in the last few years had organized resistance to
the program. We were getting bad publicity in the paper.
The community had set up an organization called "Moth-
ers' Patrols" which patrolled the Village of Central Islip
and even the hospital grounds to try to find out what was
happening, to prevent assaults on children, which, of
course, had not occurred and were not happening.

Hysteria gripped the community, and I was, frankly,
afraid that we were going to have to go back to the old
days of the closed program.

Fortunately, in my absence, the Commissioner had
made arrangements for Dave Garroway's TV show, "Today," to be put on at the hospital. After I got back Garroway asked what we should do about emphasizing the open
ward program. We suggested that they put these vocal op-
ponents—who were actually hysterical in their attitude,
telling untruths about the program and distorting it—we
suggested that he put them on his show and interview
them.

He did that, and everyone of them immediately
changed their tune and supported the program! From that
day to this, we have had no trouble. Our program is widely
accepted, and we have the full support of our
community.[10]

Dr. Bertram Brown, Director, National Institute of Mental
Health, stated that his "professional appraisal of the Milbank Memorial Fund's great impact on mental health in the United States in a wide
variety of fields includes its tremendous effect on the development of
community mental health services in the United States. Particularly
the opening of the mental hospitals and geographic decentralization
emphasized the way in which mental hospitals can serve useful community functions other than the custodial functions.

"To some extent the 1963 message of the President to Congress
which led to the important mental health center legislation can be
traced to some of the concepts and experiences which were presented

in the Milbank Memorial Fund publications. The copies of those publications in the National Institute of Mental Health library are worn and dog eared from the staff's intensive reading of them and even now in 1973 they are still found of enormous interest and value by our staff."[11]

At the same time, Dr. Morton Kramer, Chief, Division of Biometry and Epidemiology of the National Institute of Mental Health, said that, when he lectures on the history of mental disorder epidemiology, he always finds himself emphasizing the contributions of the Milbank Memorial Fund in the 1950s, the beginning of family health studies conducted by those associated with the Fund in Baltimore's Eastern Health District, and the field station studies reported in the Fund's round tables in Syracuse and Stirling County. A classic study concerned with psychiatric morbidity in families was that by Jean Downes and Katherine Simon, "Characteristics of Psychoneurotic Patients and Their Families as Revealed in a General Morbidity Study," published by the *Milbank Memorial Fund Quarterly* in January 1954.[12] The Fund provided stimulus and guidance to the Mental Health Unit of the World Health Organization at an early point in its planning of an international program on the epidemiology of mental disorders and psychiatric statistics. Of particular importance was the Fund's assistance in the planning of and participation in the Joint Technical Meeting on Epidemiological Method in Psychiatry, held in London in September 1958. This meeting was devoted to critical review of a draft monograph by D.D. Reid on *Epidemiological Methods in the Study of Mental Disorders*. Following this meeting, Professor Reid completed the Monograph which was published as No. 2 in the W.H.O. Series of Public Health Papers (1960). Subsequently, the W.H.O. initiated an extensive epidemiological program which included activities devoted to standardization of psychiatric diagnosis, revision of the section on mental disorders of the International Classification of Diseases, a nine-country pilot study of schizophrenia, and provision of technical assistance to member states on the development of programs for epidemiological research on the mental disorders and for psychiatric statistics for use in planning and evaluating programs for the control of these disorders and for training personnel in the use of quantitative methods.[13]

After the Annual Conference of 1959, the Fund organized a small Arden House Conference on the subject of the causes of mental disorders, which was to be a review of epidemiological knowledge. Several outstanding students of mental health were asked "to prepare eight review articles summarizing the present state of knowledge about different kinds of causes which had been thought to lead to mental disorders."[14]

The papers were circulated to sixteen participants in advance of the conference, and discussion openers were assigned for each paper. In their Foreword to the *Proceedings*, Ernest Gruenberg and Matthew Huxley state:

"The viewpoint implicit behind the discussions reported here is that the application of scientific methods to the problems of mental disorder will lead us to the development of effective preventive methods. No particular theory or viewpoint about the nature of mental disorders or their causes is expounded here. What will be found is a critical appraisal of established knowledge regarding the distribution of mental disorders in populations . . . . No proposals, however, will be found which attempt to translate these appraisals into action programs to affect the amount of mental disorder occurring at the present time."[15] However, during this same time Dr. Gruenberg was chairing the American Public Health Association's Program Area Committee on Mental Health and it was preparing the *Guide to the Control of Mental Disorders* which was published in 1962, transforming these technical appraisals into program objectives for mental disorder control.

During the 1961 Annual Conference—the last one that Dr. Boudreau directed—a round table was held on the topic of decentralization of psychiatric services and continuity of care. "At this round table leaders of state mental hospitals and of community mental health programs met together for a day and a half to review the present trend of state mental hospitals to decentralize their functions, to identify more closely with the communities they serve and to extend their services into the community . . . . However, therapeutic optimism regarding certain types of mentally disordered patients has been accompanied by therapeutic pessimism regarding those patients thought suitable for mental hospital care. This has led to a sharp separation of local psychiatric services from the services of the mental hospitals. Yet with modern methods of patient care a larger and larger proportion of patients who need the mental hospital at times, need community services too. Thus the round table reflects a growing awareness on the part of psychiatrists in both mental hospitals and in community mental health programs that the two systems of medical care need to be brought into closer working relationship in the interest of providing better clinical services to patients."[16]

At the time of that Conference Dr. Boudreau was 74 years of age and serving as chairman of a comittee to search for his successor. Dr. Kruse, in 1952, had resigned to assume the chairmanship of the Public Health Committee of the New York Academy of Medicine. Dr. Gruenberg left the Fund in 1961 to be the first incumbent in a new research professorship created by the Foundations Fund for Research in Psychiatry at Columbia University. Dr. Leighton was then completing his study of Stirling County. Several members of the staff felt that Dr. Boudreau regretted the Fund's failure to accomplish more in the field of mental health. He had particularly hoped that, with the development of county mental health services, the Fund would be able to devise and test a method to evaluate the impact of these services on the mental health of a given county. For various reasons, this program could not be fully implemented before his retirement.

However, before Dr. Boudreau's resignation, in 1959, a project known as the Dutchess County Program had begun. A grant to Hudson River State Hospital paid for the extra costs involved in creating a geographically decentralized unit and bringing that unit into closer contact with local resources. Simultaneously, the technical staff inaugurated evaluation research under Dr. Gruenberg's direction. After 1961, a grant was given to Dr. Gruenberg at Columbia University for its completion. As described by Dr. Gruenberg, "The evaluation studies in Dutchess County were conducted by the Milbank Memorial Fund in collaboration with others. The Hudson River State Hospital under the direction of Dr. Robert C. Hunt until 1962 and since then under the direction of Dr. Herman B. Snow, has been a crucial and consistent collaborator."[17] Essentially, the study was designed to evaluate the effect of modernizing the delivery of psychiatric services to patients from Dutchess County. "The Dutchess County Unit was set up within Hudson River State Hospital in January 1960, to provide a comprehensive and integrated treatment service for the mentally ill of Dutchess County. The concepts underlying this emphasis on decentralized, integrated, small, open and community-centered services providing flexible and continuous care can be traced through a series of Milbank Memorial Fund conferences. The participants believed that this type of service represented a needed change from traditional patterns, one which would result in better and more humane care for the psychiatrically ill, improved acceptance of mental illness by families and the community . . . . "[18] And, even more important, it might reduce the frequency of long-term, very severe social disability.

Results of the Dutchess County study were presented as part of the program on "Evaluating the Effectiveness of Mental Health Services," a round table held in connection with the Sixtieth Anniversary Conference (1965) of the Milbank Memorial Fund. The authors were still cautious in their evaluation of the program. But, by 1967, a larger body of data had been carefully examined and Drs. Gruenberg, Snow, and Bennett could report that during the first three years of the demonstration services the annual incidence of chronic social breakdown syndrome (the most severe forms of psychiatric deterioration) had declined at least 50 percent in the county served. The program prevented at least 40 man years of severe handicap per 100,000 population served each year that the new program was in operation.[19]

The Dutchess County evaluation was only one of four evaluations discussed at the 1965 Conference. The remainder evaluated mental health services carried out by other groups in other areas.

Dr. Boudreau, who had retired in 1962 after twenty-five years with the Fund, suffered a stroke on 28 January 1965 and was unable to attend the Fund's Sixtieth Anniversary Conference. The *Proceedings* include a letter of appreciation addressed to Dr. Boudreau with the signatures of the participants at the round table on evaluating the effectiveness of mental health services.

Dr. Bertram Brown (at the time of this writing, Director, National Institute of Mental Health) and Dr. Morton Kramer (Chief, Biometry and Epidemiology Division, National Institute of Mental Health) co-chaired the 1965 meeting. Dr. Brown recently said that their participation in this meeting made it possible for them to give the kind of leadership which "helped move the country's mental health coverage to the point where one-third of the nation has funded mental health centers and a million people receive care in services developed since that conference in 1965."[20]

Philip Hallen had recently been appointed President of the Falk Medical Fund in Pittsburgh and also attended the 1965 conference. He recently said that the Falk Medical Fund's program was profoundly affected by the fact that the Milbank Memorial Fund was phasing out its mental health program at a time when the Falk Medical Fund was beginning to set out its program goals and that this "affected the work of the Falk Fund immensely." They picked up some of the goals of training mental health administrators, but did not pursue the epidemiological interests which Dr. Boudreau had successfully launched.[21] So the evaluation studies of the demonstration which Dr. Boudreau began were completed even after he had retired, and their influence was still being felt many years after his death.

In summary, it might be said that Dr. Boudreau's major innovations at the Fund were his introduction of nutrition and mental health as topics for research and problems for concern. His previous work with the League of Nations helped to strengthen the international outlook of the Milbank Memorial Fund. During the prewar and World War II eras, he was actively concerned with civilian and military problems of nutrition in the United States and Canada. In the war and early postwar periods, he was closely associated with several international organizations which dealt with problems of refugees, international health, and the establishment of foundations for a lasting peace. He helped to plan F.A.O. and W.H.O. and to choose the first directors of both.

Throughout his twenty-five years at the Fund, Dr. Boudeau continued the Fund's traditional concern with population. Arriving at the Fund less than a year after its agreement to help in establishing the Office of Population Research at Princeton University, he witnessed and aided that office's development into an outstanding center for research and training in the field of demography. He also furthered the development of the Fund's own work in population, which included sponsorship of the Indianapolis Study of Social and Psychological Factors Affecting Fertility; staff cooperation with the Bureau of the Census and the Social Science Research Council in preparing a 1950 census monograph on fertility, and, with the Bureau and the A.P.H.A., in preparing a similar monograph relating to the 1960 census period; the regular publication of articles on population submitted by outsiders as well as staff; and the regular inclusion of a round table on population at the Fund's Annual Conferences.

The grants made by the Fund during Dr. Boudreau's directorship reflect his special interests in nutrition, population, housing, mental health, and world organizations, as well as his loyalty and that of the Directors to the Fund's traditional interests. Typical recipients of the grants included the Institute of Nutritional Sciences at Columbia University, the Office of Population Research at Princeton University, Cornell University for the Stirling County study of the role of environment in psychiatric disorders, and the World Federation for Mental Health.

Dr. Boudreau died 14 February 1970. Mrs. Frank G. Boudreau and her children chose the Library of the New York Academy of Medicine as repository for Dr. Boudreau's personal and scientific papers. In announcing the opening exhibit of these papers, on 19 April 1973, the Academy justly described Dr. Boudreau as *"World Physician."*

# References

[1] John G. Winant twice served as Governor of Hew Hampshire: 1924–26 and 1930–34. He was Deputy Director of the International Labor Office in Geneva, during 1934–35 and 1937–38, and Director, 1939–40. He helped to plan the U.S. Social Security Act and, in August 1935, was named as the first Chairman of the Social Security Board. He held the positions of U.S. Ambassador to Great Britain, 1941–46, and U.S. member of the Economic and Social Council of the United Nations, March-December, 1946. On 3 November 1947 he took his own life at Concord, New Hampshire. See *National Cyclopaedia of American Biography* (New York: James T. White & Company, 1953) Vol. 38, pp. 80–81.

[2] In actual fact, however, Dr. Boudreau agreed to the initiation of several later studies in the field of family planning, including the studies by Beebe in Logan County, West Virginia, and the Study of Social and Psychological Factors Affecting Fertility. See C. V. Kiser, "The Work of the Milbank Memorial Fund in Population Since 1928," *The Milbank Memorial Fund Quarterly* 49 (Part 2, October 1971): 15–62.

[3] See C. V. Kiser, *op. cit.*, pp. 15–62.

[4] H. D. Kruse, "Results of Recent Research in Nutrition," *Proceedings of the Conference on Convalescent Care,* _____ (New York: New York Academy of Medicine, 1940), p. 15.

[5] *Ibid.*, p. 22.

[6] For more details, see C. V. Kiser, "The History of the Work of the Milbank Memorial Fund in Population Since 1928," *The Milbank Memorial Fund Quarterly* 49 (Part 2, October 1971): 15–62.

[7] Samuel R. Milbank became a member of the Board 5 April 1934. He was elected Vice-President 27 April 1950 and President 21 May 1952. In 1956, when the Executive Director, Frank G. Boudreau, was elevated to the presidency, Mr. Milbank served as Chairman of the Board. He is still Chairman of the Board and, during 1962–70, he served both as President and Chairman of the Board. The new Executive Director, Dr. L. E. Burney, was elected President and Executive Director 10 December 1970, effective 1 January 1971.

[8] *The Elements of a Community Mental Health Program* (New York: Milbank Memorial Fund, 1956), p. 7.

[9] For a list of members, see *Programs for Community Mental Health* (New York: Milbank Memorial Fund, 1957), pp. 221–222.

[10] *Steps in the Development of Integrated Psychiatric Services* (New York: Milbank Memorial Fund, 1960). See also *An Approach to the Prevention of Disability from Chronic Psychoses: The Open Mental Hospital Within the Community* (New York: Milbank Memorial Fund, 1958).

[11] Dr. Bertram Brown, Personal communication, 1973.

[12] Jean Downes and Katherine Simon, "Characteristics of Psychoneurotic Patients and Their Families as Revealed in a General Morbidity Study," *The Milbank Memorial Fund Quarterly* 32 (January 1954): 42–64.

[13] Dr. Morton Kramer, Personal communication, 1974.

[14] *Causes of Mental Disorders: A Review of Epidemiological Knowledge, 1958* (New York: Milbank Memorial Fund, 1961). The statements were prepared by Jan A. Book; Brian MacMahon and James M. Sowa; George James; John H. Cumming; Donald D. Reid; H. Warren Dunham; H. B. M. Murphy; and Alexander Leighton and Jane M. Hughes.

[15] *Ibid.*, p. 7.

[16] F. G. Boudreau and E. M. Gruenberg, "Foreword", *Decentralization of Psychiatric Services and Continuity of Care* (New York: Milbank Memorial Fund, 1962), p. 5.

[17] Ernest M. Gruenberg, "Acknowledgements," *Evaluating the Effectiveness of Mental Health Services, The Milbank Memorial Fund Quarterly* 44 (Part 2, January 1966): 123.

[18] Sydney Brandon and Ernest M. Gruenberg, "Measurement of the Incidence of Chronic Severe Social Breakdown Syndrome. Has the Dutchess County Service been

associated with a Decline in Incidence?" *Evaluating the Effectiveness of Mental Health Services, The Milbank Memorial Fund Quarterly* 44 (Part 2, January 1966): 131.

[19] Ernest M. Gruenberg, Herman B. Snow, and Courtenay L. Bennett, "Preventing the Social Breakdown Syndrome," in Fredrick C. Redlich (ed.), *Social Psychiatry* (Baltimore, Williams & Wilkins Co., 1969; A.R.N.M.D. Res. Pub. 47:179–195, 1969).

[20] Dr. Bertram Brown, *op. cit.*

[21] Philip Hallen, Personal communication, 1973.

Chapter 5

# The Regime of Alexander Robertson, 1962–1969

ALEXANDER ROBERTSON was born in Dukinfield, England, 28 April 1926. Reared principally in Scotland, where his father was a practicing physician, he graduated in medicine (M.B., Ch.B.) at the University of Edinburgh in 1949. He received the Diploma in Public Health from the London School of Hygiene and Tropical Medicine in 1955 and taught there until 1958.

In that year Dr. Robertson was appointed to the Medical School at the University of Saskatchewan, Canada, where he became professor and chairman of the Department of Social and Preventive Medicine. Together with some of his colleagues, he became involved in controversies over medical care which eventually led to a 23-day doctors' strike in Saskatchewan during July of 1962.[1]

Dr. Robertson had applied for and received modest grants from the Milbank Memorial Fund covering preceptorships, travel, and teaching experiences for some of his students in preventive medicine, for the years 1959–61. He frequently recalled sitting on one of the green leather chairs in the reception room of the Fund's office, at 40 Wall Street, waiting until Dr. Boudreau could see him.

Apparently Dr. Boudreau took a liking to the young professor of preventive medicine from Saskatoon. He not only favored, in 1961, an additional grant for support of some research activities in the Department but also, later that year, recommended to the Board that Dr. Robertson succeed him as Executive Director.

Apparently, Dr. Robertson's former teacher at the London School of Hygiene, Dr. James Mackintosh, was privy to certain discussions regarding the possibility of inviting Dr. Robertson to become

91

Executive Director of the Fund. (Dr. Mackintosh, who had been oc-
cupied at the Fund during 1961–62 in writing some reports on medical and health affairs in England, had received a grant from the Fund
for this purpose.)

Dr. Mackintosh occasionally dropped into my office for a chat.
Once, during the fall of 1961, he asked me whether I knew Dr. Alexander Robertson; I told him I did not. His reply was that Dr. Robertson was a former student of his, then at the University of Saskatchewan, and that he was "a man to watch."

Shortly thereafter, as Secretary and recorder of the minutes during a special meeting of the Technical Board held at the Plaza Hotel
in December 1961, the writer noted that one of the invited guests was
Dr. Alexander Robertson of the University of Saskatchewan. At this
meeting, there was shown a documentary movie of Dr. Alexander
Leighton and his team in their exploratory survey of mental health in
several villages in Nigeria. During the ensuing discussion, Dr. Robertson offered a brief comment. Afterward it was learned that the visitor
from Saskatchewan would succeed Dr. Boudreau as Executive Director, 1 July 1962.

Dr. Robertson attached high value to the formalization of procedure and routine. He held the view that work procedures became more
efficient and less arduous if they are handled in this manner. After the
office procedures were worked out,[2] Dr. Robertson turned his attention to the *Milbank Memorial Fund Quarterly*. The *Quarterly* was giv-
en a new cover design and typographic format, and plans were made,
in 1964, to add occasional supplements (Parts Two), which would include Conference proceedings and book-length publications.[3] An Editorial Board which met at three-month intervals was formally organized, to consider acceptance or rejection of articles submitted for
publication.

Much of Dr. Robertson's initial year at the Fund was devoted to
consideration and discussions of policy and programs. Having served
as Chairman of a Department of Preventive Medicine, Dr. Robertson
was primarily interested in this field and in the general field of medical education. As the several grants that he had previously received
from the Fund suggested, he was also concerned with the professional
advancement of promising students of preventive medicine and of-

fered them opportunities for travel and widening of professional contacts.

Although these interests did indeed become elements of Dr. Robertson's program at the Fund, there were at least two other important features. One of these was the continuation of his Saskatchewan efforts to utilize the social and behavioral sciences in preventive medicine. On his initial visit to the Fund after accepting the position as Executive Director, he announced that Dr. Robin F. Badgley, a medical sociologist at the University of Saskatchewan, would join the Fund's staff within a year.

The other important feature was his interest in Latin America. This may well have developed after he joined the Fund. The Fund had long had something of an international orientation, so the decision to focus sharply on Latin America after Dr. Robertson's arrival was, perhaps, simply a change of concentration in an existing international outlook.

## Policy and Program

Working closely with the members of the Board and especially with Chairman Samuel R. Milbank, Dr. Robertson had ready for the 1963 Conference the broad outlines of a proposed policy and program for the Fund.

> The Fund retains a degree of active interest in the fields with which it has long been concerned: demography, nutrition, mental health, and general public health. The Fund is, however, more concerned with education and training projects than with research projects. It is particularly concerned with educational programs which are designed to produce men and women in the health professions able to apply their scientific knowledge to the needs of society as a whole.

> The Fund welcomes proposals from those responsible for the education of men and women in the health professions whose primary concern is with the social and preventive aspects of medicine.

## ACTIVITIES ABROAD

Throughout its history the Fund has maintained an occasional interest in work abroad, but until recently this represented but a very small part of either its professional efforts or its financial expenditure.

Largely following the lead of the pioneer work done by private Foundations in the past, the United States Government now provides immense financial resources for health research of all kinds in this country. Very large voluntary agencies spend huge sums upon the same purposes. Even in education and training, although not quite so well endowed, this country enjoys the benefit of great resources which make the contribution of a relatively small Foundation less valuable than in the past. Furthermore, governments at all levels are able and willing today, as they were not in the past, to undertake experiment and innovation.

But there are vast areas of the world without these financial resources, including the countries of Latin America. These countries are faced by many of the same problems by which North America and Western Europe were faced in the past. While more knowledge exists with which to solve the problems of health, welfare, and education today, financial support and skill in applying and extending knowledge are commonly absent.

For these reasons the Milbank Memorial Fund, although it will be continuing its activities in the United States, has accepted an increasing responsibility to join with governments, with international agencies and with other Foundations which have long operated outside the United States, in helping certain projects and programs abroad. The comparatively limited resources of the Fund, and its small staff, call for a high degree of selectivity and work abroad is almost entirely confined to the Americas.

In the countries of Latin America, where social and economic changes are so rapid, the need for health services to relate closely to the society which they serve is particularly pressing. Attempts to reproduce in heavily populated, low income, rural areas of Latin America the kinds of health, welfare and education service which have evolved in the metropolitan areas of North America and Western Europe are irrelevant and doomed to failure. Experiment with and study of health, welfare and education needs, which take into account social, economic and demographic circumstance, are in short supply, as are the personnel at all levels required to man the services which may evolve. The Fund is therefore interested in the support of educational activities abroad which are designed to satisfy the current and future needs of the societies in which those activities are taking place.[4]

In keeping with the announced change in policy, the use of the term "Division of Research" was discontinued. The "Fund Staff" was subdivided into the Office of the Executive Director, the Technical Staff, the Publications Staff, and the Administrative Staff.

The Technical Board was increased in size, and new appointments to it were drawn largely from the fields of preventive medicine and social science.

The annual conferences became, in fact, biennial conferences, and they were oriented to the new substantive interest in preventive medicine, to the new interest in social science as an approach to health problems, and to the new interest in Latin America. Round tables on demography were continued, but these were related to problems of health and demography in Latin America.

Like his predecessor, Dr. Robertson was never primarily interested in demography, population, or family planning. Again like his predecessor, however, he saw the relevance of these subjects to public health and preventive medicine. Thus, at his suggestion the Fund, in company with several other foundations, supported the strengthening of studies in population and family planning at schools of medicine and public health in Latin America. Together with officials of the other foundations, he subsequently witnessed the emergence of a strong leadership in family planning and population policy from the ranks of Latin American health professionals.

## Milbank Faculty Fellowship Program

The core of the Fund's program as developed by Dr. Robertson
was the Milbank Faculty Fellowship Program. Although this was inspired by, and to some extent patterned after, the Markle Fellowships,
in its modified form it appeared almost uniquely designed to implement the Fund's new policy and program. (The Milbank Faculty Fellowship Program is described in detail in the booklet, *The Milbank
Memorial Fund: Faculty Fellowship Program* (New York: Milbank
Memorial Fund, 1963).

The basic plan was that, during each year, 1964–1968 inclusive,
a maximum of 10 Fellows were to be appointed annually for a five-
year period. Hence the program would have a duration of five years
with respect to appointment of new Fellows, but the total duration of
the program would be ten years. The prospective Fellows were to be
nominated by the deans or equivalent officials of the schools.

According to the first announcement:

> Milbank Faculty Fellowships are available for the support
> of junior faculty members of outstanding ability, in
> Schools of Medicine and related training institutions in the
> Americas, who, having completed their basic training, have
> competence in one of the following subjects:
>
> | | |
> |---|---|
> | Anthropology | Mental Health |
> | Demography | Nutrition |
> | Economics | Preventive Medicine |
> | Environmental Medicine | Public Health |
> | Epidemiology | Social Medicine |
> | General Medicine | Sociology |
>
> and are seeking to establish themselves in full-time academic
> careers.
>
> The Fellowship will take the form of a grant to the in-
> stitution concerned, of up to $40,000, expendable over a
> five-year period upon any of the activities of the Fellow or
> of his institution which may be approved by the Fund as
> being likely to contribute to his academic growth, such as:
> —Support towards the development of teaching facilities;
> —Support towards the cost of the Fellow's research work;

—Travel to study at other centers where research or teaching in his field is in progress, or to certain scientific meetings, with the proviso that in general no Fellow shall spend more than one academic year in a center other than his own during the tenure of the Fellowship, and that any such study be approved by the Fund;

—A supplement to the Fellow's salary, which itself would be paid by the institution.

A maximum of 10 Milbank Faculty Fellowships will be available each year.[5]

The original Fellowship announcement did not spell out the specific objectives of the program; it was concerned more with mechanics than with philosophy.

When the program began, the specific objectives most frequently mentioned were "accelerated career development" and "development of leadership." After a year, however, much was also being said about "development of a cadre of leaders favorable to preventive medicine." In fact, in 1968 on their own initiative, the Fellows organized themselves into an "Association of Milbank Faculty Fellows"—one of whose aims was to promote the principles of preventive medicine.

A report on the program, published in 1968, contains the statement:

The long-term goal of the Milbank Faculty Fellowship Program is to provide for better qualified teachers of social and preventive medicine. The specific objectives are:

1.–To aid promising young educators in schools of medicine or related institutions in their professional development.

2.–To strengthen the ties between medicine and social science, the medical profession and the community and the curative and preventive aspects of medicine.

3.–To combine financial assistance with technical aid.[6]

After the Faculty Fellowship Program had begun, the Fund employed two authorities in the field of education to serve as consultants to the program. These were Dr. Per G. Stensland, of the Department of Education at the University of Saskatchewan, and Dr. Lowell Levin, Professor of Health Education at Yale. Their first duties were to help in providing technical services to the Fellows. As experts in educational theory with special experience in problems of medical education, they had the assignment of organizing seminars and workshops among the Fellows, as well as serving in the role of resource personnel to help with the solution of individual problems that might arise.

In 1967, Dr. Stensland accepted an invitation to join the staff of the Fund as a Senior Member of the Technical Staff. In this capacity, he assisted actively in the selection process, a task from which, as a consultant, he had been explicitly exempt. He was also given increasing responsibility for the day-to-day administrative aspects of the Fellowship program.

Dr. Robin Badgley left the Fund in 1968 to take on the duties of professor and director of the Department of Behavioral Science at the School of Medicine of the University of Toronto. Dr. Stensland became Dr. Robertson's principal aide insofar as the Fellowship program was concerned.

In addition to the $8,000 per year[7] alloted to each Fellow, other advantages of a Fellowship were dollars for special travel and the privilege of inviting members of the Fund's Technical Staff, Technical Board, or other experts to visit the candidate's school for lectures, seminars, and consultation. Several seminars to which all Fellows were invited (with the Fund, directly or indirectly, assuming their travel expenses) were held in various countries of Latin America. In these instances the "host" Fellow and his staff presented his own Department or School as a "case" for study and discussion. At the annual meetings of the A.P.H.A. during 1964–68, special lunches, cocktail parties, and seminars were held for Fellows in attendance. Seminars for the Fellows were arranged in London and Belgrade in 1969 and in Mexico City in 1972.

Dr. Robertson also managed to involve the members of the Board of Directors in the selection process. Potential Fellows whose candidacies survived the site visits of members of the staff and Technical Board were invited to a Selection Conference early in May at Fund headquarters. The candidates, individually and in small groups, were interviewed by panels made up of members of the Senior Staff and the Board of Directors. A dinner at the Century Club or at the Union Club was the occasion for announcing the list of candidates finally selected as Fellows of a given class. With justifiable pride Dr. Robertson noted that every member of the Board of Directors attended the dinner following the first Selection Conference.

A further potential benefit to Fellows began in 196, with the announcement that a limited number of Milbank Faculty Associate Fellowships would become available. A Fellow of three or more years' standing would be eligible to nominate a colleague to serve as Associate Fellow, at a stipend of $5,000 per year for a period of three years. A total of three Associates were appointed in 1967, five in 1969, and six in 1970.

In 1969, Dr. Robertson left the Fund to accept a position with P.A.H.O.-W.H.O. for the purpose of helping to develop a health program in the West Indies for which the Fund provided substantial support. The preceding year had been the last in which a group of Milbank Faculty Fellows had been selected; Dr. Robertson had not participated in the process because of an extended illness.

Dr. Robertson's was a vibrant personality. His energetic disposition had resulted in a liking for travel. The Milbank Faculty Fellowship program provided opportunity for much "study-travel" within the Americas—not only for him, but for senior members of the staff and for some members of the Technical Board. He prepared his trips carefully and impressed upon others the importance of careful advance preparations for their trips.

A veritable dynamo, Dr. Robertson frequently used his dictaphone at home, in the evenings, and on weekends. The dictaphone always accompanied him on trips, and his return was frequently preceded by packages of tapes returned via air mail. He worked hard and expected his staff to do the same; however, he was unusually considerate of them with respect to matters of salary and career development. For brilliant young medical students and social scientists with a bent for preventive medicine he had an especially warm heart. During his seven-year stewardship, the Fund became an acknowledged leader in the fields of epidemiology, preventive medicine, and medical education. His special interest in Latin America and the Caribbean helped, in recent years, to bring remarkable progress in public health and demography in those areas.

An evaluation of the Milbank Faculty Fellowship Program by Per G. Stensland, Lowell S. Levin, and Richard V. Kasius has recently been published. The writer would agree, in principle, with the statement made by Dr. Ronald B. Szczypkowski, who had studied the Milbank Faculty Fellowship Program for part of his recent doctoral dissertation:

> . . . clearly, the Milbank Faculty Fellowship Program encouraged a more imaginative use of money to help the person and his department professionally.
>
> Certainly the fact that the Pan American Health Organization was sufficiently impressed with the program to finance an independent evaluation study of the Milbank Faculty Fellowship Program is evidence that the program was highly considered by others. In addition, the Public Health Service Training Grants in Preventive Medicine were influenced to some extent by the Millbank Program. The former Executive Director recalled that the administrators of that program consulted him frequently before that program was launched. Again, the fact that the Faculty Fellows gave generally high ratings to many of the components of the program seem [sic] to indicate that, from their standpoint, their individual objectives were aided substantially by the Fellowship Program. All of these factors tend to give credence to the belief that the Milbank Faculty Fellowship Program made some substantial contributions to the field of social and preventive medicine and as a demonstration project showing imaginative ways of giving fellowships.[8]

The grants made during Dr. Robertson's directorship strongly reflect his interests in preventive medicine, the behavioral sciences, medical education, the fellowship program, and Latin America. There were substantial grants to the Pan American Health Organization and to the Association of Medical Schools in Colombia. Grants for experiments in the teaching of preventive medicine in the United States and other countries of the Americas were steadily increased. One of the last of this type to be inspired by Dr. Robertson was a grant to the Yale University School of Medicine on behalf of Dr. George Silver and the Urban Coalition Task Force on Health.

## References

[1] See R. F. Badgley and S. Wolfe, *Doctors Strike* (New York: Atherton Press, 1967), p. 34.

[2] Several months after Dr. Robertson's arrival, the Fund moved from the forty-ninth to the fifty-ninth floor of 40 Wall Street, because central air conditioning was available at the new location.

[3] Hitherto, the proceedings were published separately or were assembled by publishing the constituent papers in the *Quarterly* and then collating the reprints.

[4] *The Milbank Memorial Fund: Organization Policy and Program* (New York: Milbank Memorial Fund, 1963), pp. 8—10.

[5] *The Milbank Memorial Fund: Faculty Fellowship Program* (New York: Milbank Memorial Fund, 1963), pp. 5—6.

[6] *The Milbank Faculty Fellows, 1964—1973* (New York: Milbank Memorial Fund, 1968), p. 7.

[7] Several Fellows, who did not especially need the stipend of the Fellowship, received a smaller amount.

[8] Ronald B. Szczypkowski, "The Participation of Philanthropic Foundations in Continuing Professional Education." Doctor of Education dissertation, Teachers College, Columbia University, 1971. Unpublished, pp. 163—164.

# Chapter 6

# The Interregnum of 1969–1970

ALEXANDER ROBERTSON'S RETIREMENT as Executive Director and Vice President for Scientific Affairs of the Milbank Memorial Fund, effective 1 January 1970, was announced 14 May 1969. Although the announcement was made some seven months prior to the effective date, Dr. Robertson had accumulated vacation time which entitled him to leave before the end of the year. Furthermore, he had already committed himself to help in arranging seminars for selected Milbank Faculty Fellows in London and Belgrade in the summer of 1969. He actually left the office 1 July 1969. However, he did plan to return to the Fund for the October 1969 Conference on Demographic Aspects of the Black Community.

Early in May 1969, Alexander Robertson and John S. Baugh, Secretary and Vice President for Administration, visited the writer's office for an informal discussion. They had recently talked with Samuel R. Milbank, President and Chairman of the Board of Directors of the Milbank Memorial Fund, and they brought the news that there would be no immediate appointment of an Executive Director to succeed Dr. Robertson. Until such an appointment was made, the affairs of the Fund were to be in the hands of a Technical Committee, composed of three staff members of the Fund: the Vice President for Administration and the two Senior Members of the Technical Staff (Per G. Stensland and the writer, each of whom would bear the title of Vice President for Technical Affairs). The writer was asked whether he would be willing to serve as a member of the Technical Committee, and also whether, if invited, he would agree to serve as Chairman during its existence. Under this arrangement, John S. Baugh would continue in charge of Administration, Per G. Stensland would have charge of the Milbank Faculty Fellowship Program, and the writer, as Chairman of the Technical Committee, would assume responsibility for the remaining scientific or technical duties of the Executive Director. These duties would include calling meetings of the Technical Committee to consider appeals, acting as chairman of the Technical Board, and serving as chairman of the Editorial Board of the *Milbank Memorial Fund Quarterly*.

The writer told Robertson and Baugh that he would gladly undertake the duties described if asked to do so although he previously worked in the area of research rather than administration. The offer presented a challenge and, in fact, seemed to clarify the writer's position in the immediate future. Only a few days earlier he had informed Dr. Robertson that he would reach sixty-five years of age on 22 July 1969. Evidently thinking the writer was one or two years younger, Dr. Robertson had expressed surprise and agreed to talk with Mr. Milbank about the possibility of an extension, since appointments of employees sixty-five or more years of age are on an annual basis.

At the May 1969 Technical Board meeting, Mr. Milbank cordially confirmed the plans described and these were duly authorized by the Board of Directors two days later.

During his last month at the office (June 1969), Dr. Robertson cooperated wholeheartedly in the transfer of his duties to the Technical Committee. He sat long hours with the members considering, case by case, the status of existing grants and pending appeals, offering advice when asked; he discussed with the Technical Committee the record of each Milbank Faculty Fellow; he began immediately to delegate incoming appeals and letters concerning Fund matters to the Technical Committee.

The Technical Committee worked together quite well. Although the three members had separate areas of primary responsibility, each of them regularly submitted problems in his area for discussion by the Committee. John Baugh frequently referred to the full Committee problems of personnel and administrative procedure. Per Stensland frequently asked that problems relating to Milbank Faculty Fellows be placed on the agenda. The writer frequently discussed with his colleagues matters concerning the Technical Board, the Conference of

October 1969, and other problems. Each habitually invited the others to attend interviews with prospective visitors who had been given appointments, particularly if the visitor's proposal seemed to be of potential interest to the Fund. Meetings of the Technical Committee were generally scheduled for Mondays. However, special meetings were often called on short notice, and each member of the Technical Committee felt free to visit the others' offices when special problems arose.

The main part of the Technical Committee's cooperative work was the handling of the daily mail's flow of appeals for grants. Traditionally, the Executive Director of the Fund, as is true of most foundations, sifts the appeals himself or has a qualified assistant to do the first screening for him. By tradition, he himself has the authority to reject an appeal but not to make a grant. Approval must come from the Board. Like most foundations, perhaps, the Fund has, however, a small Executive Committee of the Board who can approve relatively small grants immediately; this is empowered to approve grants of less than $10,000. Grants approved by the Executive Committee are submitted to the next meeting of the full Board and these are rather routinely "ratified." However, as Samuel R. Milbank once put it, the possibility always exists for the Board to "rap the knuckles" of the Executive Committee.

The system devised for handling appeals functioned as follows: All appeals were, in the first instance, placed on the desk of Richard Kasius. He then wrote a brief abstract of the appeal on a form which had been developed for that purpose. The abstract forms were routed, successively, to Kiser, Stensland, and Baugh. Any of the three could immediately request and receive the original letter of appeal. Each could indicate, on the abstract form, "Reject" or "Discuss." If all three indicated "Reject," the form was returned to Mr. Kasius, who sent an appropriate letter of rejection. If any member of the Technical Committee wanted the case discussed, the appeal was placed on the agenda for the next meeting.

If the decision at the Technical Committee meeting was "Reject," the appeal was returned to Mr. Kasius, who sent the letter of rejection. If a decision was made to consider the appeal further, the opinion of a qualified member of the Technical Board was usually solicited by telephone or letter. If this opinion was favorable and the Technical Committee was still disposed to recommend the appeal, informal approval of the Chairman or Vice-Chairman of the Board of Directors was sought by visit, telephone, or mail before submitting the recommendation to the Executive Committee (if less than $10,000) or to the Board of Directors (if $10,000 or more).

The year 1969, which marked the midpoint of the ten-year Milbank Faculty Fellowship Program, witnessed the maximum number of Fellows and the maximum expenditure on the program. In addition to the full contingent of 42 Fellows, three Associate fellows appointed in 1967 were carried over and five were appointed in 1969. Six additional associate Fellowships were awarded in 1970, bringing the total to 14. Development grants in 1969 included continuation of those to such agencies as Princeton University's Office of Population Research, the Association of Medical Schools of Colombia, the Mt. Sinai School of Medicine (for development of teaching in community medicine), and the Pan American Federation of Associations of Medical Schools. New grants in 1969 included those to the Student American Medical Association, the American Council for Emigres in the Profession, the National Committee on Vital and Health Statistics, the Mt. Sinai School of Medicine (for development of teaching in medical sociology), and the Pan American Health Organization (in support of a program of human resources development in health in the Caribbean).

In addition to the above, the 1970 development grants included one to the Association of Ecuadorian Schools of Medicine and one to the Urban Coalition of New York.[1]

A highlight of 1969 for the writer was the Conference on Demographic Aspects of the Black Community. This had been planned earlier in the year as a part of the Fund's joint interest in demography and urban problems.[2] The aim of this Conference was to bring together some of the white and Negro demographers and social scientists to discuss certain Negro problems in cities such as those of urban migration, segregation, marriage, fertility, illegitimacy, family planning, and health.[3]

Dr. Robertson had already secured speakers for the October and December 1969 meetings of the Technical Board. At the October meeting, Dr. Fredrick C. Redlich, Dean of the School of Medicine at

Yale, spoke on the program at the School. At the December meeting, Dr. Joseph D. Beasley talked about his programs of family planning in Louisiana and some of the national problems in this field.

The meetings for March and May 1970, which were arranged by the Technical Committee, provided something novel. At the March meeting Dr. George Lythcott, the newly appointed Assistant Dean of the School of Medicine at Columbia University, discussed some problems of health in Harlem and his approach to these problems. At the May meeting, three representatives of the Student American Medical Association, with mod clothing and hair styles, talked about the aims and work of the Association and the proceedings of their recent conference in Washington—which the Fund had helped to support.

A special meeting of the Technical Board was held in June 1970, to enable the officers and executive council of the newly formed Association of Milbank Faculty Fellows to discuss, with several members of the Technical Board and Board of Directors, the possible future role of the Association and its relation to the Fund.

As it had previously done, the Editorial Board of the *Milbank Memorial Fund Quarterly* met some four times per year during this period. In preparation for these meetings, Larry Blaser, the Managing Editor, circulated in advance to members of this Board the papers submitted for publication and copies of the books submitted by publishers for review. Articles that had received unanimous individual approval or rejection could generally be disposed of without further discussion. There was frequently some division of opinion, however, and, consequently, frequent discussion about the advisability of publishing the papers that had been submitted.

Shortly after Robin Badgley's departure in 1968, Samuel W. Bloom was invited to become a member of the Editorial Board. After Alexander Robertson left, L. E. Burney was invited to become a member. Both dutifully read the manuscripts that were sent to them and either attended the meetings or sent their opinions by mail. Enlargement of the Board had the further advantage of affording a variety of expertise and decreasing the number of occasions on which manuscripts need be sent to outsiders for review. However, by virtue of the variety of interests represented, there were often divisions of opinion about the appropriateness of publishing certain papers. Quite properly, Dr. Burney began raising fundamental questions about the historic, current, and future mission of the *Quarterly*, and this matter continued in question even after his accession to office.

One further development during the 1969–1970 interregnum deserves mention. Largely on the initiative of Per Stensland, various members of the Technical Board or other individuals well known in public health who were living in, visiting, or passing through New York were periodically invited to lunch with the Technical Staff and to talk informally about their work or about a topic of common interest. Among the speakers were George Silver, Maurice Backett, Robert H. Ebert, Paul Densen, Kurt W. Deuschle, and Samuel Bloom.

The period of the interregnum ended with the accession of Dr. L. E. Burney as Executive Director on 1 September 1970.

## References

[1] See Annual Reports for 1969 and 1970 for complete listing of grants and amounts.

[2] Earlier, the Fund had cooperated with the National Urban Coalition by supporting Dr. George Silver's work on health care with that organization, and later by initial support of his appointment to the faculty of the School of Medicine at Yale University and by a grant to the New York Urban Coalition.

[3] Clyde V. Kiser (ed.), *Demographic Aspects of the Black Community, Milbank Memorial Fund Quarterly* 48 (Part 2, April 1970).

Chapter 7

# The Emerging Program in Health Care
## under L. E. Burney

On 1 September 1970 L. E. Burney began his duties as Executive Director of the Milbank Memorial Fund. He was born 31 December 1906 in Burney, Indiana, which had been founded by his ancestors. After taking an M.D. degree at Indiana University in 1930, Dr. Burney received the M.P.H. at Johns Hopkins in 1932. He entered the U.S. Public Health Service in 1932 and served as Surgeon General during 1956–1961. From 1961 until he became Executive Director of the Fund, Dr. Burney was Vice President for Health Sciences at Temple University. He had been a member of the Fund's Technical Board since 1 January 1957 and a member of its Board of Directors since 12 May 1966.

Dr. Burney invited a colleague at Temple University, David P. Willis, to accompany him to the Milbank Memorial Fund. Willis had taken the M.P.H. degree at the Uiiversity of Pittsburgh. Deeply interested in problems of medical care, he held the position of Assistant Vice President for Planning at the Temple University Health Sciences Center. First appointed as Senior Associate of the Technical Staff, he was named Vice President for Program Development and Evaluation at the Milbank Memorial Fund 16 May 1972.

In accordance with the Fund's established policy of finding a new focus for its programs every ten years, the Board of Directors initially requested Dr. Burney to identify and develop such a focus. The new purpose that resulted from his work is described in this statement, which appeared in 1972:

The system for the delivery of health services in the United States has been the object of intense and realistic criticism during much of the past decade, and a multitude of suggestions for its improvement have been advanced. These have included proposals for changes in the financing of health services, changes in the organization and provision of services and changes in the education and utilization of health manpower. After assessment of current opportunities for contributing to the process of change in the delivery of health services, and review of the activities of other funding agencies, both governmental and philanthropic, the Fund has elected to focus primarily upon the *consumer of health services*. Within this focus, the Fund will concentrate its efforts upon the exploration of more effective *utilization of health services by consumers,* with particular emphasis upon the acquisition and application of knowledge about the accessibility and acceptability of such services to consumers.

Studies of health care consumers and the factors influencing their utilization of the health service delivery system are particularly important, in the Fund's view, in the context of a growing national commitment to the concept of the entitlement of all citizens to adequate health care, and against the background of growing consumer concern with—and involvement in—the issues of access to health services and the definitions of adequacy and acceptability of such services.

While the production and staffing of health services, their distribution and their financing have received considerable legislative and professional emphasis, further knowledge and understanding are needed in the area of utilization on such critical issues as the following:

1. What are the consumer's expectations about standards and kinds of health services?

2. What social and cultural characteristics of consumers influence their utilization of health services, and how do these factors operate?

3. What types of sponsorship, organization and distribution of practice are likely to promote the most effective consumer utilization?

4. What is the effect of various fiscal mechanisms, including incentives and disincentives to use of specific services, on consumer utilization of the health care delivery system?

5. What factors influence the utilization of preventive services?

6. What are the implications of the concepts of "adequate" health services—a professional or provider judgment—and "acceptable" health services—a consumer judgment—and how are they to be included in a determination of minimal standards for a health care delivery system?

7. What are the determinants of patient "compliance," or the "appropriate" utilization of services once the patient has gained access to the system?

This selection of substantive issues and topics is of course illustrative only, and it is intended to be neither exclusive nor limiting. It does illustrate that the issues of consumer utilization necessarily involve reciprocal relationships with the questions of financing, organization, training and the resources of providers, and cannot be isolated from them. The Fund will support programs addressed to these reciprocal relationships when such programs give particular promise of contributing to knowledge of more effective consumer utilization. At the same time, while recognizing that consumer utilization of health services is affected not only by other aspects of the health care system but also by other sectors of the social system—for example, education and housing—the Fund intends to restrict its support to those programs bearing directly upon health services. This recognition of boundaries is not, however, intended to restrict the Fund's support to health professionals alone. Applications and proposals are invited from those in other professions including, but not limited to, law, the social sciences, social welfare, public administration and management, who wish to apply their knowledge and skills to problems within the range of the Fund's program.[1]

## The Study of Higher Education
## for Public Health

The major project, made possible by a grant of $500,000, is a study of schools of public health in the United States and Canada. Originally designated the "Milbank Memorial Fund Study of Higher Education for Public Health," the project was announced in the following press release, dated 14 June 1972:

> Doctor L. E. Burney, President of the Milbank Memorial Fund, announced today that the Fund is organizing a study of the higher education needs for Public Health. This will be a three-year study to explore and develop recommendations regarding future needs in higher education for professional persons who will devote their full time to the problems of organized public health activities as such.
>
> The purpose is to develop a plan to help meet the nation's need for knowledge and skill in identifying and understanding those factors which influence the health of the public in order that the most effective programs be developed for promoting and preserving the health of the individual and the community. The study will be conducted by a [Milbank Memorial Fund] Commission consisting of [Cecil G. Sheps, Chairman and] experts drawn from the fields of public health, higher education, public policy and related fields.

The members of the renamed Milbank Memorial Fund Commission for The Study of Higher Education for Public Health are:

Cecil G. Sheps, M.D. [Chairman]
Vice Chancellor, Health Sciences
University of North Carolina

Guillermo Arbona, M.D.
Professor of Preventive Medicine and Public Health
Department of Administration of Community Health Services
School of Public Health
University of Puerto Rico

Eugene W. Fowinkle, M.D.
Commissioner
Department of Public Health
State of Tennessee

Ernest M. Gruenberg, M.D.
Director, Psychiatric Epidemiology Research Unit
New York State Department of Mental Hygiene

Arva Jackson, M.S.W.
Assistant for Human Affairs
Governor's Office, State of Delaware

Charles V. Kidd, Ph.D.
Executive Secretary and Director of the Council on Federal
Relations
Association of American Universities

John A. Logan, D.Sc.
President
Rose-Hulman Institute of Technology

Jean Mayer, Ph.D.
Professor, Department of Nutrition
Harvard School of Public Health

George Metcalf, M.S.
Columnist, *Citizen-Advertiser*
Auburn, New York

Norton Nelson, Ph.D.
Director, Institute of Environmental Medicine
New York University Medical Center

George Pickett, M.D.
Director, San Mateo County, California, Department
of Public Health and Welfare

Reverend Paul C. Reinert, S.J.
President
St. Louis University

Frederick C. Robbins, M.D.
Dean, School of Medicine
Case Western Reserve University

Charles I. Schottland, A.B.
Professor of Social Welfare
Florence Heller Graduate School for Advanced Studies in Social
Welfare
Brandeis University

George A. Silver, M.D.
Department of Epidemiology and Public Health
Yale University School of Medicine

A special staff has been recruited and is working in Chapel Hill
under the general direction of Dr. Sheps. The staff members are Florence Kavaler, M.D., M.P.H., Study Director; Miriam Bachar, Research Associate; Alice Peery, Research Assistant; and Mary C. Jeff-
coat, Administrative Secretary.

The Fund has, in addition, furthered several other projects and
will continue to do so. It provided financial support for the reprinting
and distribution of Rorem's *Private Group Clinics,* which was originally published in 1932 as a report of the Committee on the Costs of
Medical Care.[2] The Fund also plans to publish a volume containing
most of the scientific papers of Edgar Sydenstricker; this will be edited by Richard V. Kasius.

The announced availability of Health Care Fellowships connotes
the continuation of a traditional type of expenditure within a new field
of interest.

Solutions to many of the problems relating to consumer utilization of health care services will require the knowledge and participation of scholars from disciplines other

than medicine itself. The Fund seeks to facilitate such participation by providing a limited number of fellowships for
beginning scholars at a significant point in their early career development. The fellowships should provide an opportunity for undertaking a sustained and guided experience within the field of medical care while building upon a
disciplined and focused knowledge in a related profession.
Their purpose will not be to induce such fellows to shift
from their base profession to medical care, but rather to
improve their ability to contribute to health services by
adding knowledge of the health care system to the applied
areas of their own profession.

These fellowships will be awarded in support of graduate students upon application by the faculty member under whose guidance the student would work and who
would assume responsibility for the student's health care
studies. Professions that may be included within a fellowship program of this kind are the social sciences (including
anthropology, economics, political science and sociology),
law, architecture, urban planning, journalism, social welfare, public administration, management and marketing.
This roster of professions should not be considered exhaus-
tive and inquiries are invited from other faculty concerning
such health care fellowships within their disciplines.[3]

The change in focus of interest of the Fund dictated a change in
the nature of the *Milbank Memorial Fund Quarterly*. Begun in 1923
as a house organ to communicate the progress of the New York
Health Demonstrations, the *Quarterly* developed into a scientific journal of public health and demography. It carried articles based upon
the work of the Fund's Division of Research as well as those submitted by other scholars in the two broad fields just mentioned.

Beginning with 1973, the *Quarterly* appeared in a new format,
with a new subtitle, and under a new editorial board. As explained in
the formal announcement:

It is clear today that health issues and problems are
no longer confined to or defined within the health sector
alone. A broader setting and perspective have been estab-

lished as environmental and ecological concerns have come to the fore together with rapid technological development, including the information sciences. There is now strong cross-institutional concern with the health sector of the society. Indeed, in and beyond the medical institution, the health sector has the attention of workers in economics, political science, law, sociology, industrial engineering, systems analysis, social welfare and other disciplines. . . .

The new subtitle of the *Quarterly*—Health and Society—is indicative of the new editorial orientation. The subtitle is intended to convey a concern with those interrelationships between social and health factors which yield outcomes and consequences for the public health, wanted or not, anticipated or not. . . .[4]

The *Quarterly* had previously been edited by the Fund's staff. In part because of the increased range of disciplines which the new orientation included, it was decided to transfer the editorship to an academic setting. George G. Reader, M.D., Livingston Farrand Professor and Chairman of the Department of Public Health at Cornell University Medical College, agreed to serve as Editor. The Editorial Board of the *Milbank Memorial Fund Quarterly/Health and Society* is as follows:

George G. Reader, M.D.
Livingston Farrand Professor of Public Health
Cornell University Medical College
*Editor*

Mary E. W. Goss, Ph.D.
Professor of Sociology in Medicine
Cornell University Medical College

Herbert E. Klarman, Ph.D.
Professor of Economics
Graduate School of Public Administration
New York University

Jeremy Morris, M.D.
Professor of Social Medicine
London School of Hygiene and Tropical Medicine

Max Pepper, M.D.
Professor and Chairman
Department of Community Medicine
Saint Louis University School of Medicine

Ernest W. Saward, M.D.
Professor of Social Medicine
Associate Dean of Extramural Affairs
University of Rochester School of Medicine and Dentistry

Alvin L. Schorr, M.S.W.
General Secretary
Community Service Society of New York

Herman M. Somers, Ph.D.
Professor of Politics and Public Affairs
Princeton University

Selvin Sonken, D.D.S.
Chief, Care Development Branch
Division of Dental Health
Bureau of Health Manpower Education
National Institutes of Health

Paul D. Stolley, M.D.
Associate Professor of Epidemiology
School of Hygiene and Public Health
Johns Hopkins University

Charles R. Wright, Ph.D.
Professor of Communications and Sociology
The Annenberg School of Communications
University of Pennsylvania

## East African Program in Medical Education

Medical Services International, Inc. (M.S.I.), was established in 1964 with the objective of supporting the efforts of three medical schools in East Africa to educate their own countrymen in Africa, by Africans, and relevant to the special needs and problems of the three countries of Uganda, Kenya, and Tanzania. Samuel R. Milbank joined the Board of Directors of M.S.I. in January 1965.

This objective was implemented originally through assisting, upon request, in the recruitment of faculty in the United States to occupy senior posts in several medical schools in East Africa while these were training their own nationals, and by providing "salary supplementation" to these individuals above the relatively low salaries received from the host countries to assist the American recruits to meet some of their continuing personal commitments, including educational costs for their children.

The Milbank Memorial Fund, among other granting agencies, contributed to the support of this program. The Board of Directors consisted of distinguished leaders from the health professions and interested laymen. This program continued until 1970 with an annual budget of approximately seventy thousand dollars.

In 1970, because of certain changes in the Internal Revenue Act, affecting the continued contributions of foundations to M.S.I. and because of the increasing requests from these three countries for expatriate faculty, the Board of Directors of the Milbank Memorial Fund, consistent with their traditional interest in and support of international health, assumed administrative and financial responsibility for the entire program.

The program has expanded greatly since the Fund assumed operational responsibility. This has been due to several factors: the continuing need of these three countries for senior expatriate faculty—especially since the medical schools in Kenya and Tanzania were only established in 1967—the high quality, commitment, and good adjustment of the Americans recruited; the preference of these countries for working with a foundation as contrasted to governments; and, finally, the important fact that the Fund does not limit its support to Americans. Almost half of the present twenty-three grantees are citizens of other countries, including Nigeria, Zambia, Ghana, and Canada.

In addition to assisting individual grantees, the Fund provides institutional grants to the schools to assist them in the development and strengthening of their newly established graduate programs. The objective is to train their specialists in their own countries so that their education will be consistent with and relevant to their particular needs and problems, their systems for delivering health services with emphasis upon public health and preventive medicine, and the economic, social, cultural, and political conditions which prevail.

According to Dr. L. E. Burney, President of the Milbank Memorial Fund, "the support of the Fund for this program in East Africa is unique among foundations, fulfills a vital need to these struggling young schools and is a most tangible and satisfying activity. It is especially gratifying to support an exceptionally fine group of highly qualified Americans from some of our leading medical schools who, with their families, adjust so well to the local environment, and are making an outstanding contribution in these three African medical schools as they struggle to train and develop their own Nationals for service and teaching responsibilities."

## References

[1] Milbank Memorial Fund, *Current Program Policy and Organization* (New York: Milbank Memorial Fund, 1972), pp. 9–11.

[2] C. Rufus Rorem, *Private Group Clinics*, Publication Number 8, The Committee on the Costs of Medical Care (Chicago: University of Chicago Press, 1931; reprinted, New York: Milbank Memorial Fund, 1971). The reprinted edition contains a Foreword by Edward M. Dolinsky and David P. Willis and the author's Preface to the Reprint Edition.

[3] Milbank Memorial Fund, *Current Program Policy and Organization* (New York: Milbank Memorial Fund, 1972), pp. 12–13.

[4] A Statement of Purpose, in *The Milbank Memorial Fund Quarterly/Health and Society* brochure, 1973.

Chapter 8

# Overview of the Fund's Sixty-nine Years of Activity

FOUNDATIONS, created and operated to serve social needs, are themselves subject to change. This chapter summarizes the changes in structure, methods and fields of interest of the Milbank Memorial Fund.

The structure of the Memorial Fund Association, 1905–1921, was quite simple, consisting only of a Board of Directors. There was no executive director and no staff. However, Albert G. Milbank performed the functions of an executive director, and he assigned necessary correspondence and clerical work to one of the secretaries in his law office. The only operating mechanism was the giving of grants. However, both Mrs. Anderson and Mr. Milbank assumed considerable personal responsibility for the grants. As has been stated, Mrs. Anderson's letter of 1913 to the A.I.C.P., which Mr. Milbank helped to prepare, indicated that even the early grants could not be interpreted simply as "forking over" money for other people to spend. The early grants to A.I.C.P. were, to some extent, "demonstration projects" designed to test the feasibility of certain approaches to problems of health and welfare on the Lower East Side.

The fields of interest of the Memorial Fund Association during 1905–1921 were, in large part, those of the Association for Improving the Condition of the Poor. The A.I.C.P., in fact, was one of the chief beneficiaries of grants during this early period. However, grants made to other organizations extended over the entire range of health and welfare, with particular attention to child health and welfare, tuberculosis, personal cleanliness (the public baths), and mental health.

The reorganization of the Fund in 1922 represented a radical expansion of structure and method. When in 1922 the Fund's Board of Directors decided to undertake the three large health demonstrations, they immediately authorized the election of a small Technical Board to develop the plans for the health demonstrations and a larger Advisory Council to review periodically the progress of these projects. Both technical boards and advisory councils are relative rarities in foundations and are virtually nonexistent in foundations whose activity is restricted to grants.

The Technical Board as first constituted was considerably more than an advisory group. At that time the Fund possessed no technical staff, so the Technical Board, in a sense, filled the gap. Although its first charge was to "mature the plans" for the health demonstrations, it was frequently called upon to advise on appeals and Fund policy. Furthermore, through the Secretary, the Technical Board could make recommendations to the Board of Directors. The strong position of the Technical Board is not surprising when one recalls that the original members included, in addition to John A. Kingsbury, seven first-rank experts in health and welfare with whom both Mr. Milbank and Mr. Kingsbury had been associated in their work for A.I.C.P. The Technical Board met frequently and served, in fact, rather as a "kitchen cabinet" for the Secretary.

When Edgar Sydenstricker became Scientific Director of the Fund in 1935, he curtailed the role of the Technical Board to an advisory function; later, there was also a reduction in the frequency of the Technical Board's meetings. However, by that time the health demonstrations had been completed, and there was a Division of Research with a capable Technical Staff.

The Advisory Council, which originally included, in addition to members of the Technical Board, some 27 leaders in the fields of health, education, and welfare, was established with the intent that it review periodically the progress of the health demonstrations. The occasions for the review became formalized rather quickly into the Annual Conferences of the Milbank Memorial Fund—another rare feature of foundations.

Prior to 1932, the Conferences were round table discussions of the problems and progress of the demonstrations. With the cessation of the demonstrations the original function of the Advisory Council also ceased. However, by that time the Fund's Division of Research had become well established. This division had been set up not only to attempt an evaluation of the demonstrations but to conduct research in selected areas of public health and such related fields as evaluation of public health procedures, medical care, nursing, and population. Therefore, during 1932–1936 the Annual Conferences generally featured several round tables. In 1932 there were five, each devoted to a particular aspect of the Fund's work. During this period the Conferences continued to be termed "meetings of the Advisory Council," but new faces appeared. After Edgar Sydenstricker became Scientific Director in 1935, the term Advisory Council was discontinued and "conference participants" were thereafter invited annually on an individual basis.

The *Milbank Memorial Fund Quarterly Bulletin* was initiated in 1923 as a device of the Technical Board to inform the Board of Directors and the Advisory Council about the progress of the health demonstrations. The *Quarterly* was not discontinued when the demonstrations terminated; it had already begun to serve the developing Division of Research as a means for publication of research papers. Like the Technical Board, the Advisory Council, and the Annual Conference, publication of a regular journal was a most uncommon feature of the Milbank Memorial Fund.

At this point it should be re-emphasized that these four rather unusual and long-lasting attributes of the Milbank Fund were established as means of aiding the three health demonstrations. Mr. Kingsbury probably deserves chief credit for them. The first two, the Technical Board and the Advisory Council, had their inception at the 11 May 1922 meeting of the Board of Directors. The third, the Annual Conference, followed as a natural means of implementing the function of the Advisory Council. The fourth, the *Quarterly Bulletin,* followed in 1923 as a natural medium of communication anent the health demonstrations, which later developed into a scientific journal.

In 1928, Mr. Sydenstricker contributed two further features that were rather rare in foundations at the time. One was the Division of Research; the other, the introduction of studies in population as an integral part of the Division of Research. The Division of Research (re-

fer to chapter 3) served as a means of transition from the almost
completed demonstrations to broader interests and research in public
health and related factors. These included expanded studies in public
health and tuberculosis; new studies in population, contraception,
nursing and medical care; and small-scale field surveys as a means of
collecting data.

Since a separate paper recently appeared on the Fund's work in
population,[1] relatively little has been said concerning it in this volume. According to Notestein,[2] Sydenstricker gave credit to Thomas
Cochran, a member of the Board, for providing the impetus for the
Fund's initiation of research in population and family planning. Some
members of the Board looked rather askance at the idea. The Scripps
Foundation for Research in Population Problems, established in 1922,
alone antedated the Milbank Memorial Fund in initiating work on
population.

The structure and methods of the Fund under Boudreau were essentially those developed by Kingsbury and modified by Sydenstricker. Shortly after coming to the Fund, Dr. Boudreau confided to Dr.
Ralph E. Wheeler and the writer that the Technical Board was his
"crown of thorns." Dr. Wheeler, then serving as Secretary of the
Technical Board, told the writer that Dr. Boudreau had been quick to
realize that certain members of the Technical Board were ready to
take advantage of his new position and his apparent good nature and
were "rubbing each others backs" in order to curry support for their
own projects. Dr. Boudreau managed to stop this practice forthwith
—and thereafter no member suspected him of being an easygoing
newcomer.

Several years later, Dr. Boudreau secured Albert G. Milbank's
agreement to put Technical Board membership on a three-year rota-
tion basis. To initiate the plan, existing members were divided into
three groups: those who would remain on the Board three years, two
years, and one year, respectively. With a twinkle in his eye, Dr. Boudreau reported that the three-year group thought this was a "splendid
idea," the two-year group thought it was a "good idea," and the one-
year group thought it was an "idea."

Dr. Boudreau's regime brought new fields of interest: nutrition,
housing, and mental health. These new fields and the continuing ones

of population and other aspects of public health were reflected in the Fund's projects, in its grants, and in the character of its Technical Board replacements.

The Annual Conferences continued as an outstanding feature of the Fund's work throughout Dr. Boudreau's twenty-five-year incumbency. During this time, two or three round tables were organized for each Conference, and population remained a perennial subject. Nutrition, housing, and various aspects of public health were other frequent topics during the prewar years.

Since the importance of certain aspects of these topics not only persisted but increased with the onset of defense preparations and wartime conditions, they continued to be topics for conference discussion during the prewar and war periods. (The conference was canceled in only one wartime year: 1945.) Round tables on population and nutrition, in particular, during this period featured ongoing research and projects by or for federal and international agencies.

Similarly, after the war there was a trend toward the round table topics on international or world problems, particularly in the demographic field. During this period, mental health gradually replaced nutrition as a conference topic and field of interest.

Under Dr. Alexander Robertson the Division of Research was abolished. Some research by the staff was continued, but major emphasis was placed on the new Milbank Faculty Fellowship project. Conferences were changed from annual to biennial meetings and the *Quarterly* was enlarged to include occasional supplements (Parts 2), which were used for publication of conference proceedings and for book-length reports. The grants, the fellowship program, and other projects were designed to support the new interests in medical education, preventive medicine, social science, public health demography, and Latin America. The Technical Board was increased in size, and its new members reflected these new fields of interest.

Under Dr. Burney, the Fund's new field of interest is that of health services, especially problems of the utilization of medical care. Grants are to be the chief method for promoting this field of interest, but, instead of waiting for appeals to come in, the staff will actively seek out potentially promising recipients for Fund grants and help them to develop projects and prepare appeals. The device of conferences based on a special purpose is also being used to further the Fund's interest in medical care. The *Quarterly* will continue, but the supplements have been dropped and an effort is being made to adapt the content of the *Quarterly* to the Fund's new interest. Articles are now selected by an outside Editor and Editorial Board.

Just as Dr. Robertson discontinued the use of the term "Division of Research," Dr. Burney has discontinued use of the term Technical Staff" in organizational structure—a part of the trend toward reduction of permanent staff in research and publications. However, a large, three-year study of schools of public health has been organized by the Fund; it is being conducted by a national commission under the direction of Dr. Cecil G. Sheps of the University of North Carolina. Much of the work is performed by a special staff with headquarters at Chapel Hill; the staff members are temporary employees of the Milbank Memorial Fund.

## The Board of Directors

In foundations, as in most organizations, the ultimate source of authority lies in the Board of Directors.[3] The Board decides on grants, appoints the Executive Director, passes on the appointment and discharge of professional personnel, and is responsible for the policy of the organization. It should be emphasized, however, that the Board of Directors tries to select an Executive Director whom it can trust, and on whom it can rely with the minimum of interference. If an Executive Director should be repeatedly rebuffed with respect to his recommendations, he knows that he would be wise to begin looking for another job.

When Mrs. Elizabeth Milbank Anderson turned to her cousin Albert Goodsell Milbank for advice about her growing list of charities, he suggested the formation of a foundation with a Board of Directors; the reason was that she had neither the time nor the knowledge needed to investigate all the appeals.

The list of past and current members of the Board of Directors of the Milbank Memorial Fund is presented in Appendix 4. These are shown in three groups—charter members, other past members, and current members. The five charter members included Mrs. Anderson's cousin, Albert G. Milbank, and the other four, Francis B. Kinnicutt, M.D., George L. Nichols, Edward N. Sheldon, and Harry Townsend (a physician and three lawyers), were either professional or personal associates of Mrs. Anderson or Mr. Milbank. Similarly, the five additional members appointed before Mrs. Anderson's death included Albert J. Milbank (father of Albert G. Milbank) and Dr. Charles M. Cauldwell (a relative of Mrs. Anderson), and the remaining three were professional or personal associates.

Two of the members of the Board of Directors, Albert J. Milbank and Dr. Kinnicutt, predeceased Mrs. Anderson. The surviving eight guided the Fund through the initial years of the three health demonstrations.

No further members were elected to the Board until 1928, when Chellis A. Austin was appointed to fill the vacancy created by the death of Dr. Cauldwell.

Of the ten present members of the Board, Samuel R. Milbank has had the longest tenure. Elected in 1934, he has been on the Board for 40 years.

## The Technical Board

Probably because the charter members of the Board were for the most part lawyers and businessmen, they realized the necessity of obtaining technical expertise when the three health demonstrations were planned. For this reason, the Technical Board and the Advisory Council were authorized. Examination of the list of past and present members of the Technical Board (refer to Appendix 5) indicates not only that all were technically competent but were recognized leaders in their fields. The charter membership of the Technical Board was weighted with physicians, educators, and social workers, for their task was to plan and guide the health demonstrations. Other specialists who successively entered on the scene were epidemiologists and statisticians, nutritionists, workers in mental health, medical educators, medical sociologists, and, finally, specialists in problems of medical care. Although their role has changed to that of advisors, they have always served to keep the work of the Fund on a solid scientific foundation and to suggest possible new fields for study.

The same may be said of the role of the Advisory Council. This group of 27 leaders in health, education, and welfare (exclusive of the members of the Technical Board, who were *ex officio* members of the Advisory Council) was established to review periodically the progress of the health demonstrations. The name "Advisory Council" was dropped after the demonstrations ended, but the basic idea was continued with the Annual Conference. The Annual Conference, a unique feature of the Milbank Memorial Fund, undoubtedly served to assist the technical staff by determining the validity of research findings subjected to periodic review and by suggesting new techniques and new fields for research. The Annual Conference also helped the Executive Director and the Board of Directors to make the work of the Fund more timely and significant.

## Members of the Staff

Appendix 6 lists past and present members of the Fund's professional and technical staff. Three categories of past members are used: Executive Directors, Administrative and Professional Staff, and Semi- and Junior Professionals. The concluding category is that of present members of the professional and technical staff. The total list contains eight who served 25 years or more, and ten who served from 10 to 24 years.

## The Secretaries of the Milbank Memorial Fund

Until the appointment of John A. Kingsbury, in 1922, there was no paid director of the Milbank Memorial Fund. His official title was Secretary, until his retirement in 1935. Edgar Sydenstricker, his successor, was appointed Scientific Director. Frank G. Boudreau became Executive Director on 1 April 1937 and President on 31 March 1956. Alexander Robertson was appointed Executive Director in 1962 and given the additional title Vice President for Health and Scientific Affairs in 1968. L. E. Burney became Executive Director 1 September 1970 and shortly thereafter was given the additional title of President.

This section, however, is concerned less with the "top brass" than with the three secretaries who have served as "second in command."

These were Catherine A. Doran, Helen Slane McGuire, and John S. Baugh.

Catherine A. Doran was employed by Albert G. Milbank 7 March 1921, two weeks after the death of Mrs. Anderson. She assisted in preparing for the 11 May 1921 meeting of the Board, when the proposals of the Special Committee on Organization were to be considered. The Committee had retained John A. Kingsbury to prepare an *Initial Report* on the work of the Memorial Fund Association during 1905–1921, including a classified list of grants. Miss Doran helped with the preparation of this report and with plans for the 11 May meeting.

As a result of the decisions made at the 11 May 1921 meeting, Catherine A. Doran became the first permanent employee of the Milbank Memorial Fund; Mr. Kingsbury was named as part-time consultant, for one year, to prepare recommendations for the future work of the Fund. For the first time the Milbank Memorial Fund had its own headquarters at 49 Wall Street; space had been rented in the old Atlantic Building, which also housed the law firm of Masten and Nichols with which Albert G. Milbank was affiliated.

In 1924, two years after Kingsbury's appointment as Secretary, Miss Doran was named Assistant Secretary. Bertrand Brown, who joined the Fund's staff as Editorial Assistant when the *Quarterly Bulletin* was instituted in 1923, was also listed as Assistant Secretary during 1925–1929. However, in 1929, Brown's title was changed to that of Director, Division of Publications. In that position, he served as editor of the *Milbank Memorial Fund Quarterly Bulletin* and assumed responsibility for much of the work in public relations to which Kingsbury attached more importance than did any of his successors. Miss Doran's sphere of responsibility was general administration; she kept records of the grants, paid the bills, made the physical arrangements for the meetings of the Board of Directors, the Technical Board, and the Annual Conferences, and had much of the responsibility for hiring and firing of clerical personnel. She performed these duties for Kingsbury, Sydenstricker; and Boudreau. She was named Secretary in 1937 and retired 31 December 1955.

Helen Slane McGuire began work for the Milbank Memorial Fund 30 November 1925. At the beginning, she worked mainly for

Bertrand Brown, the editor of the *Quarterly Bulletin* who also had charge of the pool of stenographers and typists. She became Frank Boudreau's private secretary when he came to the Fund in 1937 and also served as Assistant Secretary of the Fund. Succeeding Miss Doran as Secretary on 1 January 1956, she continued the tradition of efficiency established by her predecessor. She worked hard herself and succeeded in getting good productivity from her staff. With a reputation for strictness, she was always helpful, taking an interest in the welfare of everyone connected with the Fund. Having served under four directors, she retired 31 December 1968 after 43 years, a record for length of service with the Fund second only to (and just short of) that of Albert G. Milbank, who was a member of the Board of Directors for 44 years, from 1905 to 1949.

John S. Baugh came to the Milbank Memorial Fund 15 July 1968 as Secretary-elect and Vice President for Administration. Previously resident in Peru as Vice President of the International Basic Economy Corporation and Managing Director of the Negociacion Azucarera Nepena, S.A., he has devoted much attention to the fiscal affairs of the Milbank Memorial Fund, introducing economies and modern systems of budget control. By virtue of his talents and interests in financial affairs, he has taken over important functions of the treasurer that formerly were fulfilled by the United States Trust Company. His full title is Executive Vice President, Secretary and Treasurer. Because of these additional responsibilities, he needed and was given assistance in the office. Juan A. Inclan, who first joined the Fund in 1963 to serve as Alexander Robertson's Administrative Assistant, was named Supervisor of the office in 1969.

Since each Secretary has served under two or more directors, each has preserved a measure of continuity despite changes in directorship. Moreover, just as many of the day-to-day duties of the executive director devolved upon Miss Doran during the year between Sydenstricker's death and Boudreau's appointment, John Baugh similarly was a member of the Technical Committee responsible for the Fund's affairs during the interregnum of 1969–1970.

The names of most other administrative and professional members of the staff have been mentioned in earlier chapters.

## The Role of the Foundation
## in American Life

Like other institutions, foundations possess both strengths and weaknesses. Since their beginning they have been recurrently praised and criticized. In 1920, E. A. Ross, a sociologist at the University of Wisconsin wrote: "It is to be feared that foundations of ample means . . . . will in time show the unadaptedness to be expected of self-continuing boards."[4] In 1936, Eduard C. Lindeman, another sociologist, in his study of 100 foundations and community trusts, wrote of the striking tendency for members of the boards of foundations to be drawn from the "successful and conservative class" and especially from the ranks of bankers and lawyers.[5]

After World War II, a great increase in the number of small, family-sponsored foundations was followed by allegations of abuse of tax-exempt privileges. To curb these abuses, the Tax Reform Law was enacted a few years ago.

This law naturally provoked a good deal of complaint among foundation executives; no doubt it was at least partially responsible for a good deal of soul-searching on the part of foundation executives and former officials.[6] In the fall of 1972, a four-day conference was held at Arden House under the sponsorship of Columbia University American Assembly, at which trustees, directors, and other officers of large foundations attempted to reconsider their aims and the means of achieving them.[7]

There is probably considerable justification for the allegations of Ross, Lindeman, and others concerning the conservative nature of foundations in general, but two points must be made about the Fund's Board of Directors. Although the majority of the Board's members have been drawn from the fields of law and business, approximately one-third of the 37 past and present members have been physicians, educators, nutritionists, and social workers.

Furthermore, it was precisely *because* the majority of the members of the Board of Directors were not medical men that the "founding fathers" of the Fund established the Technical Board, whose members have been outstanding leaders in the health professions, and

whose specialties have reflected the changing interests of the Fund
and have helped to prevent a narrow isolationism.

Whatever their weaknesses, foundations fill several distinct roles
and possess undoubted sources of strength. They have considerably
more freedom than government agencies to initiate research or experimental action in new fields or sensitive areas. They are in a better position to take risks on research and in expenditure of funds. They can
well serve as catalysts, to "prime the pump," to provide seed money,
and to demonstrate that specific problems are areas of proper concern
for local, state, or national governments, or for other private agencies.

In the writer's view, four outstanding sources of strength possessed by foundations are (1) availability of funds—inherent in the
nature of a foundation, (2) specificity of interest, (3) quality of leadership, and (4) possibility of periodic renewal of youthful vitality by
a change of program. With respect to funds, given a definite income,
foundation officials need not include fund-raising and annual appeals
among their numerous duties and worries.

Unlike the university, where diffuse fields of interest cluster
around education, the foundation can focus its efforts sharply. As to
leadership, foundations frequently lure their executive directors from
universities, government agencies, and business firms. The position of
executive director offers the opportunity and the challenge to develop
a program within a given area—more or less according to one's wishes, a salary at least comparable to that of professors at the leading
universities, and a comparative freedom from some of the stresses
now endemic on the campus and in the market place.

The Milbank Memorial Fund has been fortunate in possessing
strong leadership. Each Executive Director has had his own particular
set of skills, talents, and interests. Although the record is not without
instance of resignation because of differences between the Director
and Board over ideas of policy or direction for the Fund, each of the
Fund's past directors served for a considerable period of time with the
firm support of the Board—and each made notable contributions.

To the author, at least, a review of the Fund's achievements during the administrations of the successive directors suggests that a major wellspring of strength of the Fund, and of other foundations, has
been the periodic changes of course. These changes, prompted by new

directors, may not be welcomed by those who have benefited under previous regimes; undoubtedly, however, they have helped to maintain a freshness of approach and a timeliness of objective—qualities which are surely needed, for today's problems inevitably differ from those of yesterday.

# References

[1] Clyde V. Kiser, "The Work of the Milbank Memorial Fund in Population Since 1928," *Forty Years of Research in Human Fertility: Retrospect and Prospect, The Milbank Memorial Fund Quarterly* 49 (Part 2, October 1971): 15–62.

[2] Frank W. Notestein, "Reminiscences: Role of Foundations, the Population Association of America, Princeton University and the United Nations in Fostering American Interest in Population Problems," *Forty Years of Research in Human Fertility. . . ,* p. 69.

[3] "The [Milbank Memorial Fund] corporation elects a Board of Directors of ten members at its annual meeting. Full power in the management and control of the business and affairs of the corporation is vested in this Board, which holds four stated meetings a year. An Executive Committee acts for the Board in the intervals between meetings." Milbank Memorial Fund, *Current Program Policy and Organization,* (New York: Milbank Memorial Fund, 1972), p. 4.

[4] E. A. Ross, *The Principles of Sociology* (New York: The Century Company, 1920), p. 313.

[5] Eduard C. Lindeman, *Wealth and Culture* (New York: Harcourt, Brace and Company, 1936), pp. 45–46.

[6] Waldemar S. Nielsen, *The Big Foundations, A Twentieth Century Fund Study* (New York: Columbia University Press, 1972).

[7] *New York Times,* 7 November 1972, p. 31.

# News Story from The New York Sun, 1903

## SHE GAVE BARNARD MILLION
## MRS. ELIZABETH M. ANDERSON
## NAME OF THE GIVER

### She Is the Daughter of the Late Jeremiah Milbank and the Wife of A. A. Anderson, the Artist —She Gave First Barnard Building Built on the New Site

The gift of $1,000,000 to Barnard College for the purchase of three city blocks immediately south of the present college buildings on Morningside Heights, which was announced by President Butler of Columbia and Treasurer Plimpton of Barnard on Friday was not made by John D. Rockefeller, as has been generally supposed, but by Mrs. Elizabeth Milbank Anderson, wife of Abram A. Anderson, a well-known artist. She is the daughter of the late Jeremiah Milbank, who died in this city in 1884 leaving about $10,000,000 to be divided between his daughter and his son, Joseph Milbank.

One of the conditions of the gift to Barnard was that, for the present, at least, the name of the donor should not be made public. In the announcement of the gift on Friday it was stated over the signatures of Dr. Butler and Mr. Plimpton that no one but themselves knew the name of the donor and that it would be kept a secret for the present.

The Sun learned, however, on the highest authority yesterday, that the $1,000,000 was offered by Mrs. Anderson, and was accepted several weeks ago, long before the public was allowed to know of Barnard's good luck.

This last gift to Barnard will make almost $2,000,000 that Mrs. Anderson and her brother, Joseph Milbank, have made to Barnard and to Teachers' College, affiliated with it. Mrs. Anderson's interest in the institution, always great, has been growing in recent years, and when she heard that the institution's development absolutely required the three city blocks south of the present buildings for the erection of a second academic building and at least two more dormitories, she set about to find out how much the property could be secured for.

The property is owned by the New York Hospital, several of the trustees of which are also trustees of Columbia, so that the negotiations were carried on in a spirit of the greatest friendliness.

It is said that after Mrs. Anderson made her offer to Barnard of $1,000,000, a price slightly in excess of that figure was fixed by the trustees of the New York Hospital. Mrs. Anderson, it is said, promptly met the advance. In round figures, however, her gift to Barnard is $1,000,000, the largest lump sum that has ever been given to the institution, and the largest lump sum ever given away by Mrs. Anderson.

Mrs. Anderson is said to have given away in the neighborhood of $3,000,000 for charitable and educational purposes in the last dozen years. She is an extremely modest giver, however, and when she can, prefers to have her gifts anonymous. Most of her large gifts for educational purposes have, like this one to Barnard, been credited to

some other person for a long time before the real giver was discovered by the general public.

Mrs. Anderson's father, Jeremiah Milbank, began his business career in this city as a grocer, and was a member of the old-time firm of I. and R. Milbank on Front Street. Some twenty years before his death, however, he retired from the grocery business and entered the financial world, opening a banking and brokerage office at 90 Broadway.

He was an extremely shrewd business man and piled up a large fortune. In 1858 he advanced the capital for the formation of the Borden Condensed Milk Company and was a heavy stockholder in it when he died in 1884. He was also a member of the executive committee of the Chicago, Milwaukee and St. Paul Railroad.

Mr. Milbank's daughter married Abram A. Anderson, the portrait painter, whose studio, said to be one of the handsomest in this country, is in the building owned by Mrs. Anderson at Fortieth street and Sixth Avenue. Mrs. Anderson has always made her city home in the old Milbank residence at 6 East Thirty-eighth Street, but she has a handsome home at Greenwich, Conn. where she spends a good deal of her time.

On November 29, 1892 Mrs. Anderson, through her lawyer, Elihu Root, offered to build a medical pavilion in memory of her father and mother, Jeremiah and Elizabeth Lake Milbank, for Roosevelt Hospital, The offer was made to the trustees of the hospital and was coupled with the condition that the building should be used only for medical clinics and should be in charge of Dr. Francis P. Kinnicutt, his successor after his death to be selected by the College of Physicians and Surgeons.

So interested was Mrs. Anderson in this gift that she sent Charles A. Rich, the architect, abroad to study foreign hospitals and get the best ideas for the kind of a building she had in mind. Her offer to the trustees was accompanied by complete plans made by Mr. Rich, and it was accepted at once.

Ground was broken for the new building, but before a stone had been laid the trustees decided that the conditions of the gift were somewhat irksome and decided to refuse it unless they were relieved of some of them. There were a number of conferences, but Mrs. Anderson stuck to her original proposition, so the gift was declined.

For this new building Mrs. Anderson had offered $350,000. When it was declined she decided to spend the money for some other useful purpose. Money, and a great deal of it, was needed for Barnard College when it moved to its new site on Morningside Heights opposite Teachers' College and the new Columbia buildings.

Mrs. Anderson had always been interested in the college and the greater part of the money she had offered to Roosevelt Hospital was used to build the first of the Barnard College buildings on the new site. This building is now known as Milbank Hall.

Shortly after Mrs. Anderson made this gift to Barnard, Teachers' College was desperately in need of funds for a new building. Joseph Milbank, Mrs. Anderson's brother, came forward, unsolicited, and give the money needed, $250,-000. This gift was said to be the result of the interest in the Morningside Heights educational institutions aroused in Mr. Milbank by his sister's gift to Barnard.

Some years ago Mrs. Anderson built a memorial hospital for a small Connecticut town, which was badly in need of such an institution, and the public baths now being erected on Thirty-eighth street, between First and Second avenues by the Society [*sic*] for Improving the Condition of the Poor are being built out of a gift of $150,000 made by Mrs. Anderson to the society for the purpose.

Outside of her charitable work, which takes up a good deal of her time, Mrs. Anderson's chief amusement is driving. She is an accomplished whip and believed by many to be the best woman driver in this city.

*The New York Sun*

Vol. LXX—No. 189, page 1.

Appendix 2

# MINUTE

## ADOPTED BY THE
## BOARD OF DIRECTORS
## OF THE
# MILBANK MEMORIAL FUND

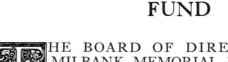HE BOARD OF DIRECTORS OF THE MILBANK MEMORIAL FUND, at a meeting held May 11, 1921, adopted the following minute in memory of Mrs. Elizabeth Milbank Anderson, at whose suggestion the association was founded and to whom it owes its entire endowment.

"Elizabeth Milbank Anderson, daughter of the late Jeremiah and Elizabeth Lake Milbank, was born in New York City December 20, 1850.

"All her life a resident of New York City, Mrs. Anderson's name is known throughout the country, and among the sick and needy of many other countries, as a generous and great-hearted woman, filled with human sympathy and eager to relieve suffering and distress among all sorts and conditions of men. She studiously avoided publicity, and many of her generous acts will never be known, but her larger gifts arrest the attention by their variety and wisdom. While perhaps her chief benefactions were in the interests of women and children, her generous impulses knew no bounds, and her gifts, often unsolicited and unexpected, cover a widely diversified range.

"To Barnard College, of which she became a Trustee in May, 1894, and Vice-Chairman of the Board in May, 1899, Mrs. Anderson gave in 1896 the Administration Building on 119th Street, known as 'Milbank Hall,' and which, together with the buildings flanking it, Fiske Hall and Brinckerhoff Hall, formed the original group in which the College was housed after it left its old site at 343 Madison Avenue, to join Columbia University on Morningside Heights.

"A little later, in 1903, Mrs. Anderson, realizing that the future of Barnard depended upon the control of sufficient property to permit of expansion, purchased of the New York Hospital, at a cost of a million dollars, the three city blocks bounded by 116th and 119th Streets, and by Broadway and Claremont Avenue, and gave this important site, now vastly more valuable than when it was purchased, to Barnard College. Since then, on this property, which is known as 'Milbank Quadrangle,' there have been constructed Brooks Hall, a College dormitory, built with funds provided by her, and Students' Hall, a gift of the late Jacob H. Schiff. She also contributed liberally and constantly to the general and special funds of the College, and was the personal friend of many of its students, who, but for her aid and encouragement, might never have been able to obtain a college education. In fact, without the immense stimulus in the institution's early years of her fruitful and earnest suggestions, supported by her munificent and far-sighted aid, Barnard College would not occupy its present notable position in the educational life of the country.

"In 1909 Mrs. Anderson gave to the Children's Aid Society the land and buildings known as 'The Home for Convalescent Children,' at Chappaqua, New York, to which are sent each year large numbers of children from the poorer sections of the city, who are either suffering from some obstinate ailment requiring prolonged treatment, or who are afflicted with the after-effects of some serious illness. At Chappaqua, with its beautiful buildings, cheery rooms and spacious grounds, thousands of waifs from the city's tenements have found health and happiness. From time to time Mrs. Anderson has made additional gifts to the Society for maintenance and as endowment for the Home, so that the total for this purpose now aggregates about a million dollars.

"For the past fifteen years she has been vitally interested in public health work and in promoting constructive measures with a view to minimizing poverty by trying to remove some of its causes. Convinced that sickness is one of the chief reasons for poverty, she gave of her strength and her money, to promote the health of the community. One of her first gifts of this kind was made to the New York Association for Improving the Condition of the Poor, in the form of the Milbank Public Bath building on East 38th Street, which was so perfect in its design and in its operation that it served as a model for the series of Municipal public baths subsequently built and maintained by the City. A few years later she became deeply concerned to learn that, for lack of funds, the organization which had been serving nourishing luncheons at a penny a portion in a few of the public schools, was about to abandon this work. Being satisfied that this service should be continued in the interests of the health of the children, she undertook to finance it herself, choosing the Association for Improving the Condition of the Poor as her medium. This resulted not only in serving the school lunches in the six or eight original schools, but the service was extended to over thirty schools, at which approximately two million lunches a year were served.

"Recently school lunches have been taken over by the City, under the management of the Board of Education, thereby making this feature a part of the Public School system. Simultaneously with the school lunch project, Mrs. Anderson made it possible for the Association for Improving the Condition of the Poor to create what is known as its Social Welfare Department, which confines itself to constructive and preventive measures in contrast to the work of relieving distress among the poor. Through Mrs. Anderson's generosity and clear vision this social welfare work now includes community health centers, dental clinics for children, and the Victoria Apartments, which is a Home Hospital, where families, with one or more tubercular members, are housèd and treated just as effectively as if the sick member had been sent to a sanitarium in the country, but with the added advantage of not breaking up the family life.

"An entirely different field, in which Mrs. Anderson has taken an active and important part, embraces the work to improve the care of the insane and mentally deficient, and to forestall the development of mental disorders. Her gifts to the National Committee for Mental Hygiene have enabled that organization to create widespread and intelligent interest in the subject, and to win a hold on public support that insured the future permanency and success of its work.

"Among negro schools of the South, among medical missionaries in China, and throughout countless educational and charitable organizations Mrs. Anderson's name and vivid personality will long be held in affectionate and grateful memory.

"During the Great War she gave unstintedly to the relief and welfare organizations, and she purchased and sent through her own organization tons of food continuously and regularly for several years, to aid the suffering people of Belgium and France, and since the armistice she has made it possible for the Memorial Fund Association to give largely to the sick and destitute children of Serbia, and for the starving children of Central Europe. In recognition of her great services to France, she was created by the Government in 1918 a chevalier of the Legion of Honour.

"To facilitate and perpetuate this broad scheme of benevolence, Mrs. Anderson, in 1905, requested five friends to associate themselves together as a membership corporation, with extensive charitable powers, and in fulfilment of this the incorporation of The Memorial Fund Association was duly completed on April 3, 1905. By deed of trust dated May 27, 1907, she transferred to the Association about three million dollars in securities, to be held in trust, to collect the income therefrom, and after applying $5,000 of such income in each year to the charitable purposes of the trustee, to pay over the balance to the creator of the trust during her lifetime. Upon her death the trust was to cease and the fund to become the absolute property of the Association. In pursuance of the power reserved by this deed, Mrs. Anderson, on April 23, 1913, transferred to the Association about $2,840,000 of additional securities, to be held upon the same trusts. In October, 1913, in order to relieve herself of the responsibility of providing financial assistance to certain projects of magnitude, the trust was modified so as to vest in the Association the power to apply to its charitable purposes so much of the income of the trust property as in the judgment of the Directors was adequate or desirable to accomplish such purposes, and to pay the balance of such income, if any, to Mrs. Anderson. A further transfer of $200,000 of securities was made by her to the Association May 23, 1916, and of $250,000 more on December 10, 1917. By an instrument dated December 12, 1918, Mrs. Anderson completed the amendment of the scheme of the original deed of trust by relinquishing all right of revocation of the instrument and any right to receive income from the fund. The entire fund thereby vested in the Association absolutely. Her last gift to the Association was made in January, 1919, and included 15,000 shares of common stock of Borden's Condensed Milk Company. The share certificates were not actually received by the Association until March 22, 1919, but were then accompanied by a check for $60,000, representing the dividend of 4% paid on the stock February 15th.

"The Association also has in certain contingencies rights in three trust funds created by Mrs. Anderson in her lifetime:

"(1)  By· a deed dated March 31, 1919, she transferred to Albert G. Milbank and the Mercantile Trust & Deposit Company (now known as the Mercantile Trust Company) $20,000 in cash and 22,500 shares of the aggregate par value of $2,250,000 of the stock of The 415 Fifth Avenue Company, Inc.  This Company is the owner, subject to a mortgage of $1,600,000, of the property known as the Bonwit Teller Building, at the southeast corner of Fifth Avenue and 38th Street, with an extension running to 37th Street.  The trust is for the life of her granddaughter, Elizabeth Milbank Anderson, Second, so much of the income to be applied to her benefit by the trustees as they deem best, and any unexpended income to be paid to the Memorial Fund Association.  After she reaches 35 years of age she is to receive not less than two-thirds of such income, and the remaining one-third will belong to this Association.  Upon her death leaving issue, the principal of the fund goes to such issue, but in default of such issue, to the Association.

"(2)  By another deed, dated March 31, 1919, Mrs. Anderson conveyed to Mr. Milbank and the Bankers Trust Company the property numbers 9 and 11 East 37th Street, now leased to the Nine East Thirty-seventh Street Company, in trust, to pay the income therefrom to her daughter, Mrs. Campbell, during her life, and on her death to convey and transfer the principal of the trust to the Memorial Fund Association.

"(3)  By a third deed, dated May 12, 1920, Mrs. Anderson conveyed to Mr. Milbank and the United States Trust Company of New York her residence known as 'Milbank' and about seventy-seven acres of surrounding land at Greenwich, Connecticut, in trust for her own benefit during her life, and on her death in trust for the benefit of her granddaughter, Elizabeth Milbank Anderson, Second.  By the terms of this deed, the trustees are vested with the broadest discretionary powers with reference to the trust property, and may convey it all at any time to the granddaughter.  If this discretion is not exercised in favor of the granddaughter, any residue of the trust estate becomes the property of the Association.

"In addition to these munificent endowments, Mrs. Anderson, by her will, which was proved in the New York Surrogates' Court March 10, 1921, made the following provisions for the Association: (1) An interest in remainder in a trust fund for $250,000 held during the life of her daughter, Eleanor Anderson Campbell; (2) an interest in remainder in a trust fund of $250,000 held in trust during the life of her granddaughter, Elizabeth Milbank Anderson, contingent upon her death without leaving issue; and (3) a general legacy of $1,500,000.

"While recognizing the value and necessity for organized charity, Mrs. Anderson was always intolerant of red tape and had no patience with organizations which emphasized form above substance; therefore it frequently happened that she indulged in what she called 'unconventional giving,' and on these occasions she revelled in the shocked surprise of the orthodox administrators of the benevolent work.

"Keen in mind, possessed of sound business judgment, with a rare sense of humor, buoyant in spirits, strong in her likes and dislikes, counting loyalty as one of the supreme qualities in human relationship, fearless and ever ready to fight for the right as she saw it, scornful of weakness and insincerity in others, she went through life a valiant soul, whose loss will be mourned by a host of people who came directly or indirectly under her influence. To the members of this Board, who knew her so well, it is a grateful duty to record here, however incompletely, this minute of her inspiring accomplishment and of our affectionate remembrance."

EDWARD W. SHELDON,
*President.*

ALBERT G. MILBANK,
*Secretary.*

Appendix 3

# Excerpts from Initial Report
# MILBANK MEMORIAL FUND

## HISTORICAL SUMMARY OF ITS ORGANIZATION
## AND DEVELOPMENT

### INTRODUCTORY SUMMARY

The Milbank Memorial Fund was founded, as "The Memorial Fund Association", at the suggestion of Mrs. Elizabeth Milbank Anderson, to whom it owes its entire endowment. The certificate of incorporation, filed and recorded April 3, 1905, was executed by Mr. Edward W. Sheldon, Mr. Howard Townsend, Dr. Francis B. Kinnicutt, Mr. George L. Nichols and Mr. Albert G. Milbank, the original Board of Directors. At a special meeting held at the home of Dr. Kinnicutt, 39 East 35th Street, on May 4, 1905, the Certificate of Incorporation was presented by the Counsel, and the Directors formally organized by adopting unanimously the proposed by-laws submitted by Counsel. Mr. Edward W. Sheldon was elected President and Mr. Albert G. Milbank Secretary and Treasurer, to serve until the first annual meeting.

ORGANIZATIO.

The original Board of Directors served without change until January 16, 1914. At this meeting Dr. Charles M. Cauldwell was elected to fill the vacancy caused by the death of Dr. Francis B. Kinnicutt. The only other change in the original Directors that has taken place was the election of Mr. John G. Milburn on December 29, 1920, to succeed Mr. Howard Townsend, who felt compelled to resign. On January 17, 1921, the number of members of the Board was increased from five to seven, and at the following meeting on January 28, 1921, Mr. Elihu Root was elected to membership, and on February 1, 1921, Mr. Thomas Cochran was chosen to fill the remaining vacancy.

At the first annual meeting Mr. Edward W. Sheldon and Mr. Albert G. Milbank were elected to succeed themselves as President, and as Secretary and

INCORPORATIO

Treasurer, respectively. These officers have succeeded themselves at each successive annual meeting, except for a period of five years during which Mr. Albert G. Milbank was relieved of the duties of Treasurer. At the meeting held May 27, 1907, Mr. Albert J. Milbank was made a member of the corporation and was elected to the office of Treasurer, which he held continuously until his death on May 23, 1912. At the meeting of June 14, 1912, Mr. Albert G. Milbank was again elected Treasurer and has continued to serve as Secretary and Treasurer up to the present time. At the meeting of May 27, 1907, Mr. George L. Nichols was elected Assistant Treasurer, which office he held until the annual meeting of January 28, 1921, when the United States Trust Company was elected Assistant Treasurer.

The certificate of incorporation sets forth the purposes for which the corporation was formed in the following language:

PURPOSES

"To further secular and religious education among all classes; to care for the sick, the young, the aged and disabled; to minister to the needs of the poor; to improve the phyical, mental and moral condition of humanity and generally to advance charitable and benevolent objects.

To extend financial or other aid or assistance to such individuals, corporations, associations or institutions as are now, or may hereafter be, engaged in furthering the purposes above named, or either of them, and to establish, promote, maintain and endow, in whole or in part, any such corporations, associations or institutions."

In furtherance of the above purposes the certificate of incorporation provides that the Memorial Fund Association "shall have power to acquire by deed, devise, bequest, gift or purchase or otherwise real and personal property, and to hold, invest, reinvest, manage and dispose of the same". It provides further that the operations of the Fund are to be principally conducted in the United States of America, and that its principal office shall be located in the City of New York.

GIFTS

During the sixteen years of its operations under the name of "The Memorial Fund Association" the Fund received from Mrs. Elizabeth Milbank Anderson gifts the par value of which amounted to

$7,815,175.  By her will Mrs. Anderson left the Fund
$1,500,000, thus increasing the entire amount of her
gifts, at par value, to a total of $9,315,175.  She ex-
pressed in her will the desire that within one year after
her death, which occurred on February 22, 1921, the
corporate name should be changed to the "Milbank
Memorial Fund".  This request was promptly complied with by resolution adopted March 30, 1921, the
action being legally effective on April 16, 1921.

Since its organization the Memorial Fund has
appropriated $1,544,504.10 to the following charitable
organizations and educational institutions, classified
according to the dominant character of their work,
which constitute the sum of the beneficiaries of the
Memorial Fund during the first sixteen years of its
corporate existence:

| Organization | Appropriation | Total |
|---|---|---|
| **Child Welfare:** | | |
| A. I. C. P. | $248,208.31 | |
| Babies' Dairy Assn. | 4.500. | |
| Babies' Welfare Assn. | 250. | |
| Boy Scouts of America | 250. | |
| Children's Aid Society | 108,037.48 | |
| Crippled Children's Fund | 1,000 | |
| Girl Scouts of America | 500. | |
| N. Y. Child Labor Committee | 10,000. | |
| State Charities Aid Assn. | 10,000. | |
| | | -$ 382,745.79 |
| **Public Health, Including Mental Hygiene:** | | |
| A. I. C. P. (Child Health) | $248,208.31 | |
| Amer. Social Hygiene Assn. | 1,000. | |
| Com. of Ref. & Council for Health | | |
| Education in China | 3,000. | |
| National Com. for Mental Hygiene | 95,000. | |
| Public Health Com. N. Y. Acad. of | | |
| Medicine | 4,000. | |
| State Charities Aid Assn. | 2,500. | |
| | | 353,708.31 |
| **General Health, Including Hospital Relief:** | | |
| A. I. C. P. (Home Hospital) | $52,000. | |
| Trudeau Sanitarium | 77,000. | |
| Fifth Ave. Hospital Bldg. Fund | 10,000. | |
| Flower Hospital | 5,000. | |
| Greenwich Hospital | 5,000. | |
| Henry Street Settlement | 50,000. | |
| National Social Unit Organization | 21,000. | |
| N. Y. Baptist Mission Society | 1,000. | |
| United Hospital Fund | 2,500. | |
| | | 223,500. |
| | Forward | 959,954.10 |

| Organization | Appropriation | Total |
|---|---|---|
| Brought forward | | $959,954.10 |

**General Relief:**

| | | |
|---|---|---|
| A. I. C. P. | $20,000. | |
| Assn. for Blind & Crippled Sailors & Soldiers | 1,000. | |
| Baptist Home for Aged | 5,000. | |
| China Famine Relief Fund | 5,000. | |
| Institute for Crippled & Disabled Men | 1,000. | |
| Legal Aid Society | 127,500. | |
| | | 159,500. |

**War Relief and War Work:**

| | | |
|---|---|---|
| Amer. Com. for Armenian & Syrian Relief | $5,000. | |
| Amer. Com. for Devastated France | 1,000. | |
| American Red Cross | 31,950. | |
| American Relief Administration | 50,000. | |
| Auto Army Service | 10,000. | |
| Commission for Relief in Belgium | 15,000. | |
| Natl. Com. of U. S. for Restoration of Univ. of Louvain | 1,000. | |
| Relief Work in France | 5,000. | |
| Salvation Army (Home Service Fund) | 1,100. | |
| Serbian Relief Com. | 5,000. | |
| Serbian Child Welfare Assn. (National Birthday Committee) | 100,000. | |
| United War Work Campaign | 10,000. | |
| Y. M. C. A. War Camp | 10,000. | |
| Y. W. C. A. Fund | 5,000. | |
| | | 250,050. |

**Education:**

| | | |
|---|---|---|
| American School in Tokio | $40,000. | |
| Barnard College | 10,000. | |
| Bryn Mawr College | 1,000. | |
| Community Council of National Defense | 2,500. | |
| Fisk University | 10,000. | |
| Grinnell College | 5,000. | |
| International Assn. of Vacation Bible Schools in Far East | 3,000. | |
| League to Enforce Peace | 5,000. | |
| Music School Settlement | 3,000. | |
| National Consumers League | 4,000. | |
| National Country Life Assn. | 5,000. | |
| N. Y. Public Library (Children's Room) | 2,500. | |
| Princeton University | 10,000. | |
| Self Government Committee | 1,750. | |
| Tuskegee Normal Industrial Institute | 25,000. | |
| Training Service for Community Workers, Columbia Univ. | 1,000. | |
| Working Women's Protective Union | 5,000. | |
| | | 133,750. |
| Forward | | 1,503,254.10 |

| Organization | Appropriation | Total |
|---|---|---|
| Brought forward | | $1,503,254.10 |

**Miscellaneous:**

| Organization | Appropriation | Total |
|---|---|---|
| Bowling Green Neighborhood Assn. | $ 150. | |
| Inter-Church World Movement | 1,000. | |
| Inter-Racial Council | 2,000. | |
| Madison Ave. Baptist Church Endowment Fund | 36,000. | |
| National Information Bureau | 500. | |
| Summer Band Concert Fund | 1,500. | |
| | | 41,250. |
| | | $1,544,504.10 |

The above classification indicates the lines of work which have most strongly commended themselves to the Directors of the Milbank Fund and points to the rather marked tendency to emphasize child welfare and public health work, including mental hygiene. This is more clearly indicated if the appropriations for war relief and war work, made as the result of a great world crisis, are eliminated from consideration. The action of the Board in making this distribution very closely follows the dominant and well known interests of the donor of the funds. Mrs. Anderson, throughout her purposeful life, always gave liberally to relief in a great emergency, although her clear preference was to support organizations interested in child welfare, especially in its preventive aspects, and those engaged in public health and preventive medicine. It is evident, therefore, that the Milbank Fund, while not crystalizing its interest into fixed policies, has shown a clear tendency to devote the major portion of its income to child welfare and public health. The wisdom of this will be clearly brought out in the analysis of the work of some of the organizations which have been the principal beneficiaries of this Fund.

## CHILD WELFARE

The organizations engaged in child welfare work to which the Milbank Fund has contributed cover a wide range of activities—child health, convalescent care, treatment of crippled children, finding homes for orphans, education, recreation and legislation for the protection of children. By far the most extensive work in the interest of children supported by the Fund is that which has been conducted by the

A.I.C.P. under its Department of Social Welfare. Indeed, the work of this Department is, in a broad sense, child health work. It is therefore somewhat difficult to determine whether it should be classified as child welfare or public health work.

When Mrs. Anderson made her large gift to the Memorial Fund in 1913, it was accepted with the understanding that certain charitable and educational contributions to which she was committed would be assumed by the Milbank Memorial Fund. The most important of these commitments is outlined in Mrs. Anderson's communication to the New York Association for Improving the Condition of the Poor, providing for the establishing of a Department of Social Welfare. This plan outlined by Mrs. Anderson is so significant and far-reaching in its scope and in the results which have grown out of it that it seems appropriate to quote the letter in full, thus indicating the nature and more particularly the spirit of the most important pledge which the Memorial Fund assumed.

DEPARTMENT<br>
OF SOCIAL<br>
WELFARE<br>
A. I. C. P.

## Letter of Gift

"March 5, 1913.

R. Fulton Cutting, Esq.,
President New York Association for
Improving the Condition of the Poor,
105 East 22nd Street, New York City.

My dear Mr. Cutting:

Pursuant to the preliminary announcement made by Mr. Milbank on my behalf at the last meeting of your Board, I beg to say, after conference with the Committee appointed by the Board, that I am prepared to finance for a period of ten years, and within certain limits, the various activities which are hereinafter summarized and which will be conducted under the supervision of a new department to be created by the Association to be known as the Department of Social Welfare.

In undertaking this matter it is perhaps well for me to indicate in a general way the objects I have in mind.

In the first place I am particularly interested in fostering preventive and constructive social measures for the welfare of the poor of this city, as distinguished from relief measures affecting particular individuals and families. I fully appreciate the necessity for ministering to the physical needs of the sick, disabled and unfortunate, but in undertaking the work outlined in this letter I wish to make it clear that the proposed Department of Social Welfare is to concern itself, in so far as it employs funds supplied by me, with a social program based upon preventive and constructive measures.

Generally speaking, therefore, this program should include those activities which are calculated to prevent sickness and thus relieve poverty, such, for example, as the promotion of cleanliness and sanitation and the securing of a proper food supply. In this connection your Association will doubtless find it advisable, in some cases, to co-operate with public authorities, and with existing agencies having similar objects in view where such agencies are practicing approved methods in fulfilling their purposes, while in other cases it may probably be necessary to establish the work as a new enterprise, and in still other cases it will perhaps be prudent to devote some time and money to investigation and research before assurances can be given that any proposed measure will accomplish the object sought to be attained.

With this general comment I would say that I will be glad to furnish the necessary funds to meet the annual expenses of operation incident to the carrying on of the proposed work, to the extent of Fifty Thousand Dollars per annum for ten years and, further, will furnish as required such amount as may be necessary up to One Hundred and Fifty Thousand Dollars to cover initial or capital charges and the cost of certain experimental and research work, which will be more particularly referred to below.

With these funds at your disposal I would expect you to create the proposed Department of Social Welfare, and to distribute the enterprises to be conducted under its supervision among at least three sub-departments or committees, one having jurisdiction over matters pertaining to Public Health and Hygiene, one having jurisdiction over matters pertaining to the welfare of School Children, and one having jurisdiction over matters pertaining to the food supply of the working classes of this City.

Under the heading of Public Health and Hygiene I would expect that the Milbank Memorial Baths in East 38th Street be maintained in its present state of efficiency as a model bath, and that an active educational campaign be carried on for the purpose of inducing the City to maintain the same standard of economy and efficiency in respect of the Baths operated by it, and for the further purpose of demonstrating to the City the advisability of extending the Public Bath System in properly selected sections of the City, and generally to popularize the public bathing facilities so as to increase their usefulness to the utmost. Under this heading also I would favor equipping one of the present typical floating baths with a modern and approved filtering device, which I am advised can be made available and which would eliminate the present chief objection to the floating baths as now conducted. As a sub-division of this same heading I would favor making a careful study of the present conditions in New York in regard to Public Comfort stations and in connection therewith the formulation of a program for extending this system and for maintaining a higher standard of cleanliness and sanitation in these places. Another sub-division under this heading would consist in investigating the subject of Public Laundries, and, if feasible, the establishment of such a laundry, preferably in connection with the 38th Street Baths, but if this is not feasible then at some other suitable location. It is well known that the facilities for doing laundry work in the homes of the poor are most inadequate and in many cases are absolutely lacking, with the result that it is very difficult, if not impossible, for the poor to maintain a healthful standard of personal cleanliness. Experience in other cities has shown that such a service is eagerly availed of and, so far as its cost of operation is concerned, can be made self-supporting. Such laundries, I am informed, are in successful operation in London and other European centers, and in some cities in this country, but no effort in this direction is being attempted in New York. And here again the idea would be to demonstrate by a model laundry the practicability and the desirability of establishing similar but public laundries throughout the city, possibly in connection with the city bath houses.

Under the heading of Public Health and Hygiene would also fall such an allied activity as the promotion of a campaign to exterminate as far as possible the house fly, and other similar carriers of disease and thereby minimize the danger to the public health from such sources. I understand efforts in this direction, meeting with a considerable degree of success, have been made in various localities, but so far as I know no well organized contiuous effort of this kind has as yet been made in New York. I consider this a very important matter and trust that it will be given proper attention. In this connection, as also in other lines, it would be wise to consider the advisability of securing the assistance of an auxiliary committee made up of persons especially interested in this subject and which would carry out an educational program under the supervision of the Association.

Under the heading of the Welfare of School Children I would expect that the admirable work for some years last past conducted by the School Lunch Committee (which I am informed is about to disband), would be broadened and continued under the supervision of your Association. This is a matter in which

I would like you to avail yourselves of the experience
and interest of the existing School Lunch Committee,
or at least of such members thereof as are available.
I would wish, however, to have this feature of the work
broadened when placed under your control, so that it
would furnish lunches to the children of a group of
approximately fourteen Public Schools, to be selected
with the idea of benefiting those most sorely in need of
proper nourishment, and at the same time with a view
to improving upon the methods heretofore employed, by
establishing one or more central kitchens from which
the lunches would be conveyed in wagons to the various
schools, as is now done by one of the leading restaurant
companies in the City. It has been calculated that for
the amount of money at your disposal for this feature
of the work approximately six hundred thousand lunches can be served during the school year for which a
charge of only one cent a portion would be made. It
is gratifying to realize that by utilizing the service of
the present School Lunch Committee, it will be possible
to have this branch of the work organized and in operation by the time the schools open in the Autumn. It
is my hope that by continuing this enterprise as a model
unit embracing approximately fourteen schools, the
system may be extended to such extent as may be
needed either by other individuals or organizations, or
by the City, as a part of the Public School system.

In connection with this enterprise I would like an
enquiry to be made regarding the feasibility of establishing a Public Bake Shop, to which those who have
no facilities for baking bread or roasting meats could
bring their uncooked food and at a nominal cost receive
the benefit of this service. Under existing conditions
the poor as a rule are compelled to cook most of their
food on the tops of ordinary stoves, with the result
that the food is not as healthful or as nouishing as it
should be. Furthermore, it is calculated that there
would be a substantial saving to them in the cost of
preparing their food if they had the benefit of a central
cooking plant. I understand this idea has never been
attempted in this country, but is in successful operation abroad.

Under this same heading there should be inaugurated a program for extending and improving the present system of making medical inspection of school
children, and therein co-operating with existing organizations interested in this work, and particularly with
the City Departments which have jurisdiction over matters of this kind. Closely analogous to this feature of
the work would be the attempt to increase the Clinic
facilities for the treatment of the physical defects of the
children disclosed by such medical inspection, and
particularly Dental Clinics, as it seems to be widely
recognized that the school children not only suffer very

generally from defective teeth but also that many of their ailments are due to that cause.

Under this heading would also fall an existing evil in our public schools by seeking to induce the City to intall in each school sanitary drinking fountains, instal-ling, if necessary, in one school such a device in order to illustrate its desirability. So also it would be well to secure the installation of an approved sanitary system of cleaning the school rooms in one of the school build-ings, with the idea of inducing the City to abandon its present unsanitary methods.

Under this same heading I intended to speak of the matter of proper school ventilation, but information re-ceived from your committees has persuaded me to be-lieve that the subject of ventilation as applied to places of public gathering is one which requires further re-search and experimentation, and I will therefore refer to it again as a separate matter.

Under the heading of the Food Supply to the poor I have only certain general ideas to suggest at this time, realizing that the subject is one of great complexity and that it will take much time and thought to work out the proper ways and means to accomplish the desired result. Generally speaking, however, an investigation should be made concerning the scientific production of food, it purchase in wholesale quantities, its scientific storage, its efficient and honest handling, and the latest facts as to relative food values should be brought to-gether with the object of ascertaining whether the cost of food cannot be reduced to the consumer, its nourish-ing qualities increased, and at the same time yield a reasonable return on the capital invested. I would have no sympathy with any attempt to usurp in the name of Charity the field of legitimate business. On the other hand, if investigation showed that the cost of food to the poor was excessive by reason, for example, of the use of false weights and measures, or by the abuse of the facilities of the cold storage plants, or by the adul-teration of food products, or by uneconomical methods of handling, or by unconscionable or over many profits, I would consider that a very different situation was pre-sented, and that such evils would justify your Associa-tion in establishing, for example, a People's store or market, to demonstrate that the business could be con-ducted successfully and on an honest basis. It is poss-ible that the Co-Operative Store idea might suggest the solution of this problem. As I said before, however, the subject is not sufficently clearly understood at pre-sent, to determine just what method is advisable to re-duce the cost of living to the poor, and at the same time to improve the quality of their food, but I am hopeful that a thorough investigation will result in a clearer understanding of the facts.

In conclusion, I refer to the subject of ventilation

more especially as it applies to the Public Schools of New York, in which my interest is particularly keen, but also more broadly as it applies to all places of public gathering. I am told that there are certain fundamental facts which are not clearly understood by the experts who have made a study of the subject and that a very considerable amount of research work and experimentation will be required to be done before these facts are ascertained.    Under these circumstances I am willing to allow such amount as may be necessary up to Fifty Thousand Dollars out of the One Hundred and Fifty Thousand Dollars above referred to, to be devoted to the expenses incident to this work of research and experimentation in the matter of ventilation, provided your Association will undertake to secure the services of a committee of recognized experts who will agree to donate sufficient of their time in an effort to solve this problem.    I understand that certain leading experts in this subject have signified their willingness to serve on such a committee without remuneration because of the value, both to the cause of Science and that of Humanity, that would result from their labors.    I also understand that they estimate that this research work may of necessity continue for as long as four years, and the estimated cost of $50,000. is figured on that basis.    If, however, the results are obtained in less time, the full amount of the estimate would, of course, not be required.

I would suggest that provision be made for the keeping of separate accounts on your books in relation to expenditure of these funds and also to the publication thereof.

While expressing in this letter my personal wishes and also the views of the Special Committee of your Board so far as made known to me, the acceptance of my proposal is not intended to bind your Association to a literal adherence to those wishes in case future experience shall, after conference with me or with my representative, lead your Board to the conviction that the plan heretofore set forth ought to be modified.

If it shall at any time seem to your Board desirable to extend to the Boroughs of the Bronx, Queens and Richmond any of the activities or studies herein described, and if it shall be deemed feasible to do so within the limits of my gift, I should heartily approve of such extension.

Upon receiving word that your Association is prepared to undertake this matter along the lines indicated in this letter, I will be ready to furnish the necessary funds from time to time as they may be required.

I am,

Yours very sincerely,

ELIZABETH MILBANK ANDERSON."

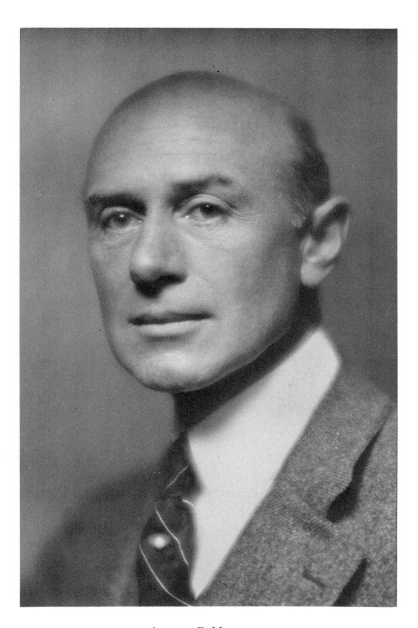

ALBERT G. MILBANK

## Appendix 4

## Members, Board of Directors, Milbank Memorial Fund, 1905 to Present

| Name | Occupation | Affiliation | Date Elected | Date of Termination | | Number of Years on Board |
|------|-----------|-------------|--------------|------|------|-------|
| | | | | By Retirement | By Death | |
| **Charter Members** | | | | | | |
| Albert G. Milbank | lawyer | Senior Partner, Milbank, Tweed, Hope and Webb; Chairman of the Board, Borden's | 2/18/05 | | 9/7/49 | 45 |
| Francis B. Kinnicutt, M.D. | physician | Professor of Clinical Medicine, Columbia University | 2/18/05 | | 5/2/13 | 8 |
| George L. Nichols | lawyer | Masten and Nichols | 2/18/05 | 1/7/30 | | 25 |
| Edward W. Sheldon | banker and lawyer | President, U.S. Trust Company of New York | 2/18/05 | | 2/14/34 | 29 |
| Howard Townsend | lawyer | President, New York State Hospital for Consumptives | 2/18/05 | 12/29/20 | | 16 |
| **Other Past Members** | | | | | | |
| Albert J. Milbank | businessman | Treasurer, New York Condensed Milk Co. (Borden's) | 5/27/07 | | 5/23/12 | 5 |

| Name | Occupation | Position / Firm | | | | No. |
|---|---|---|---|---|---|---|
| Charles M. Cauldwell, M.D. | physician | | 1/1/14 | | | 14 |
| John G. Milburn | lawyer | Carter, Ledyard & Milburn | 12/29/20 | | 1/17/28 | 10 |
| Elihu Root | statesman | Secretary of War (McKinley Administration); Secretary of State (T. Roosevelt Administration) | 1/28/21 | 5/27/30 | 8/11/30 | 9 |
| Thomas Cochran | banker | Partner, J. P. Morgan Co. | 2/1/21 | | 10/29/36 | 16 |
| Chellis A. Austin | banker | President, Seaboard National Bank | 3/26/28 | | 12/13/29 | 2 |
| Frank L. Polk | lawyer | Davis, Polk, Wardwell | 1/7/30 | | 1/7/43 | 13 |
| Linsly R. Williams, M.D. | physician | Managing Director, New York Academy of Medicine | 1/7/30 | | 1/1/34 | 4 |
| Roland S. Morris | lawyer | (in private practice) | 5/27/30 | | 11/23/45 | 15 |
| Cornelius N. Bliss | merchant and financier | Director, Bliss, Fabyan & Co.; President, A.I.C.P. | 10/21/30 | | 4/5/49 | 18 |
| Livingston Farrand, M.D. | college president | President, Cornell University | 4/5/34 | | | 6 |
| Barklie M. Henry | businessman | Former Director, A.I.C.P. | 4/5/34 | 1/20/63 | 11/8/39 | 29 |
| John A. Kingsbury | foundation executive | Secretary, Milbank Memorial Fund | 4/5/34 | 4/18/35 | | 1 |
| Franklin B. Kirkbride | investment counsel | (private firm) | 4/5/34 | | 9/28/55 | 21 |
| James G. Affleck, Jr. | lawyer | Milbank, Tweed, Hope & Webb | 4/19/35<br>4/15/47 | 6/19/37<br>5/12/66 | | 2<br>19 |

### Other Past Members

| Name | Occupation | Affiliation | Date Elected | Date of Termination | | Number of Years on Board |
|---|---|---|---|---|---|---|
| | | | | By Retirement | By Death | |
| Morris Hadley | lawyer | Partner, Milbank, Tweed, Hadley & McCloy | 6/18/37 | 5/13/65 | | 28 |
| Beekman Hoppin Pool | social work executive | State Charities Aid | 6/18/37 | 5/6/42 | | 5 |
| George A. Sloan | industrial executive | Various firms; also, President, The Nutrition Foundation | 10/15/43 | 5/5/55 | | 12 |
| Frederick H. Osborn | businessman and demographer | Treasurer, American Eugenics Society | 3/12/46 | 3/14/63 | | 17 |
| Frank G. Boudreau, M.D. | foundation executive | President, Milbank Memorial Fund | 3/21/56 | 5/31/62 | | 6 |
| Dean A. Clark, M.D. | physician | Director, Massachusetts General Hospital | 3/21/56 | 3/8/62 | | 6 |
| C. Glen King, Ph.D. | biochemist | President, The Nutrition Foundation, Columbia University | 5/9/63 | 5/16/72 | | 9 |
| Cornelius N. Bliss, Jr. | businessman | Wood, Struthers & Winthrop | 10/21/49 | 5/21/74 | | 25 |

### Current Members

| Name | Occupation | Description | Date | |
|---|---|---|---|---|
| Samuel R. Milbank | investment banker | Chairman, Board of Directors, Milbank Memorial Fund; Partner, Wood, Struthers & Winthrop; President, Pine Street Fund | 4/5/34 | 40 |
| George Baehr, M.D. | physician | Former Medical Director, H.I.P. | 12/20/46 | 2.7 |
| Charles E. Saltzman | investment banker | Partner, Goldman, Sachs & Co. | 4/27/50 | 24 |
| Thomas I. Parkinson, Jr. | businessman | (private firm) | 3/8/62 | 12 |
| Francis H. Musselman | lawyer | Milbank, Tweed, Hadley & McCloy | 5/10/62 | 12 |
| R. Bruce McBratney | businessman | Wood, Struthers & Winthrop | 12/10/64 | 9 |
| Alexander D. Forger | lawyer | Milbank, Tweed, Hadley & McCloy | 12/9/65 | 8 |
| L. E. Burney, M.D. | foundation executive | President and Executive Director, Milbank Memorial Fund | 5/12/66 | 8 |
| Robert H. Ebert, M.D. | academician | Dean, Harvard Medical School | 5/16/72 | 2 |
| Samuel L. Milbank | businessman | Salomon Brothers | 5/21/74 | 0 |

Appendix 5

## Members of the Technical Board of the Milbank Memorial Fund, 1922 to Present

| Name | Affiliation | Dates of Appointment | | Length of Appointment (Nearest Year) |
|------|-------------|------|------|------|
| | | From | To | |
| **Charter Members** | | | | |
| Herman H. Biggs, M.D. | Commissioner of Health, New York State | 5/22/22 | 6/28/23* | 1 |
| Bailey B. Burritt | General Director, A.I.C.P. | 5/22/22 | 12/31/46 | 25 |
| Homer Folks | Secretary, State Charities Aid Association | 5/22/22 | 12/31/46 | 25 |
| James Alexander Miller, M.D. | President, New York Tuberculosis Association | 5/22/22 | 12/31/47 | 26 |
| Linsly R. Williams, M.D. | Deputy Commissioner of Health New York State; Director, National Tuberculosis Association | 5/22/22 | 1/8/34* | 12 |
| William H. Welch, M.D. | Dean, School of Hygiene and Public Health, Johns Hopkins University | 5/22/22 | 4/30/34* | 12 |
| Livingston Farrand, M.D. | President, Cornell University | 5/22/22 | 11/8/39* | 17 |
| John A. Kingsbury | Secretary, Milbank Memorial Fund | 5/22/22 | 4/18/35 | 13 |

## Other Past Members

| | | | | |
|---|---|---|---|---|
| Matthias Nicoll, Jr., M.D. | Commissioner of Health, New York State | 11/19/23 | 3/20/30 | 6 |
| Thomas J. Parran, Jr., M.D. | Commissioner of Health, New York State; Surgeon General, U.S. Public Health Service | 11/25/20<br>4/5/34 | 4/29/33<br>12/31/62 | 1 |
| Shirley W. Wynne, M.D. | Commissioner of Health, New York City | 12/20/32 | 12/31/33 | 1 |
| John H. Wyckoff, M.D. | Dean, School of Medicine New York University | 10/26/34 | 6/1/37* | 3 |
| Wade Hampton Frost, M.D. | Professor of Epidemiology (Formerly Dean), School of Hygiene and Public Health, Johns Hopkins University | 3/20/36 | 4/1/38* | 2 |
| Lowell J. Reed, Ph.D. | Professor of Biostatistics (later President), Johns Hopkins University | 3/20/36 | 4/28/66*** | 30 |
| Edward S. Godfrey, Jr., M.D. | Commissioner of Health New York State | 12/19/41 | 12/31/47 | 6 |
| C.-E. A. Winslow, M.D. | Professor of Public Health, Yale University School of Medicine | 12/15/44<br>3/21/51 | 12/31/47<br>1/8/57* | 9 |
| Ernest L. Stebbins, M.D. | Commissioner of Health, New York City | 12/21/45 | 12/31/46 | 1 |
| Dean A. Clark, M.D. | Director, Massachusetts General Hospital | 12/20/46 | 4/30/63** | 16 |
| Rowland Burnstan, Ph.D. | Secretary, State Charities Aid Association | 12/19/47 | 12/31/50 | 3 |
| Harry S. Mustard, M.D. | Commissioner of Health, New York City | 12/19/47 | 7/1/55 | 8 |
| Herman E. Hilleboe, M.D. | Commissioner of Health, New York State | 12/17/48 | 4/30/69 | 21 |
| Leonard A. Scheele, M.D. | Surgeon General, U.S. Public Health Service | 12/16/49 | 12/31/56 | 7 |
| Thomas A. C. Rennie, M.D. | Director, National Association for Mental Health | 10/19/55 | 5/21/56* | 1 |

* Appointment terminated by death   ** Consultant during part of the term of service

| Name | Affiliation | Dates of Appointment From | To | Length of Appointment (Nearest Year) |
|---|---|---|---|---|
| | Other Past Members | | | |
| Paul H. Hoch, M.D. | Commissioner, New York State Department of Mental Health | 5/17/56 | 12/31/63 | 8 |
| Robert C. Hunt, M.D. | Assistant Commissioner for Community Mental Health Service, New York State | 12/16/59 | 12/31/63 | 4 |
| Frank G. Boudreau, M.D. | Retired President, Milbank Memorial Fund | 7/1/62 | 2/14/70* | 8 |
| Ernest M. Gruenberg, M.D. | Professor of Phychiatry, Columbia University College of Physicians and Surgeons | 5/9/63 | 4/30/68 | 5 |
| Henry van Zile Hyde, M.D. | Director, Division of International Medical Education, A.A.M.C. | 5/9/63 | 4/30/66 | 3 |
| C. Glen King, Ph.D. | President, The Nutrition Foundation, and Associate Director, Institute of Nutrition Sciences, Columbia University Medical Center | 5/9/63 | 5/31/72 | 9 |
| Colin M. MacLeod, M.D. | Deputy Director, Office of Science and Technology, Office of the President, U.S.A. | 5/9/63 | 4/20/66 | 3 |
| J. Wendell Macleod, M.D. | Executive Director, The Association of Canadian Medical colleges | 5/9/63 | 5/13/71 | 8 |
| Anthony M.-M. Payne, M.D. | Chairman, Department of Epidemiology and Public Health, Yale University | 5/13/65 | 4/30/70* | 5 |

| Name | Position | | | |
|------|----------|---|---|---|
| Paul M. Densen, D.Sc. | Deputy Commissioner of Health, New York City Department of Health | 10/14/65 | 4/30/70 | 5 |
| William H. Stewart, M.D. | Surgeon General, U.S. Public Health Service | 10/14/65 | 4/30/69 | 4 |
| Samuel W. Bloom, Ph.D. | Professor of Community Medicine, Mt. Sinai School of Medicine | 5/1/67 | 5/13/71 | 4 |
| Howard J. Brown, M.D. | Health Services Administrator and Commissioner of Health, New York City | 10/13/66 | 4/30/68 | 2 |
| Jack Elinson, Ph.D. | Professor of Administrative Medicine, Columbia University School of Public Health and Administrative Medicine | 10/13/66 | 4/30/70 | 4 |
| Maurice E. Backett, M.D. | Professor, Department of Community Health, University of Nottingham, England | 10/10/67 | 5/13/71 | 4 |
| Paul J. Sanazaro, M.D. | Chief, National Center for Health Services Research and Development, Health Services and Mental Health Administration | 5/13/71 | 5/31/72 | 1 |
| James G. Haughton, M.D. | Executive Director, Cook County Hospital, Chicago | 5/13/71 | 6/30/72 | 1 |
| Eveline M. Burns, Ph.D. | Professor Emeritus, New York School of Social Work, Columbia University | 8/12/71 | 8/31/73 | 2 |
| Kurt W. Deuschle, M.D. | Professor and Chairman, Department of Community Medicine, Mt. Sinai School of Medicine | 5/1/69 | 5/31/74 | 5 |
| Herman M. Somers, Ph.D. | Professor of Politics and Public Affairs, Princeton University | 5/13/71 | 5/31/74 | 3 |

* Appointment terminated by death

| Name | Current Affiliation | Dates of Appointment From | Dates of Appointment To | Length of Appointment (Nearest Year) |
|---|---|---|---|---|
| | **Members** | | | |
| George Baehr, M.D. | Special Medical Consultant, Health Insurance Plan of Greater New York | 12/17/37 | Present** | 36 |
| L. E. Burney, M.D., Chairman | President, Milbank Memorial Fund | 12/19/56 | Present | 17 |
| Rustin McIntosh, M.D. | Professor Emeritus of Pediatrics, Columbia University College of Physicians and Surgeons | 12/19/56 | Present | 17 |
| Abraham Horwitz, M.D. | Director, Pan American Health Organization | 5/1/63 | Present | 11 |
| George A. Silver, M.D. | Professor of Public Health, Yale University School of Medicine | 5/9/63 | Present | 11 |
| Robert H. Ebert, M.D. | Dean, Harvard Medical School | 5/12/66 | Present | 8 |
| Alvin L. Schorr, M.S.W. | General Director, Community Service Society, New York | 5/13/71 | Present | 3 |
| Ernest W. Saward, M.D. | Professor of Social Medicine and of Medicine and Associate Dean for Extramural Affairs, University of Rochester, School of Medicine and Dentistry | 8/12/71 | Present | 3 |

| | | | | |
|---|---|---|---|---|
| Mack Irwin Shanholtz, M.D. | Commissioner of Health, Commonwealth of Virginia | 6/1/73 | Present | 1 |
| Robert M. Sigmond, M.A. | Executive Vice President, Albert Einstein Medical Center, Philadelphia | 6/1/73 | Present | 1 |
| Arva D. Jackson, M.S.W. | Regional Equal Employment Opportunity Officer, Department of Health, Education, and Welfare, Region III, Philadelphia | 6/1/73 | Present | 1 |
| Herman B. Wells, LL.D. | Chancellor, Indiana University | 6/1/73 | Present | 1 |
| Howard N. Newman, M.B.A., J.D. | President, Dartmouth-Hitchcock Medical Center, Hanover, New Hampshire | 6/1/74 | Present | 0 |
| Edward B. Perrin, Ph.D. | Director, National Center for Health Statistics, Department of Health, Education, and Welfare | 6/1/74 | Present | 0 |

\* Appointment terminated by death       \*\* Consultant during part of the term of service

Appendix 6

## Past and Present Professional and Technical Staff of the Milbank Memorial Fund

| Name | Title at Retirement | Dates of Service From | Dates of Service To | Years of Service (Nearest Year) |
|---|---|---|---|---|
| **Past Executive Directors** | | | | |
| John A. Kingsbury | Secretary | 5/11/22 | 9/18/35 | 13 |
| Edgar Sydenstricker | Scientific Director | 1/1/26 | 3/19/36 | 10 |
| Frank G. Boudreau | President | 4/1/37 | 7/1/62 | 25 |
| Alexander Robertson | Executive Director and Vice President for Health and Scientific Affairs | 7/1/62 | 12/31/69 | 7 |
| **Past Administrative and Professional Staff** | | | | |
| Catherine A. Doran | Secretary | 3/7/21 | 12/31/55 | 35 |
| Bertrand Brown | Director, Division of Publications | 4/15/23 | 12/31/33 | 11 |
| Helen S. McGuire | Secretary | 11/30/25 | 12/31/68 | 43 |
| Jean Downes | Member, Technical Staff | 10/11/26 | 3/31/58 | 31 |

| Name | Title | | | |
|---|---|---|---|---|
| Dorothy G. Wiehl | Senior Member, Technical Staff | 10/26/26 | 12/31/63 | 37 |
| Frank W. Notestein | In Charge, Population Studies | 10/1/28 | 9/30/36 | 8 |
| Marian G. Randall | Member, Technical Staff | 9/1/29 | 12/31/37 | 8 |
| Clyde V. Kiser | Vice President for Technical Affairs | 10/15/31 | 12/31/70 | 39 |
| Margaret W. Bernard | Research Associate | 2/1/32 | 1/31/34 | 2 |
| Regine K. Stix | Member, Technical Staff | 6/1/32 | 8/31/41 | 9 |
| Ralph E. Wheeler | Member, Technical Staff | 8/1/32 | 2/15/39 | 7 |
| Isidore S. Falk | Research Associate | 1/1/33 | 12/31/35 | 3 |
| Harry D. Kruse | Member, Technical Staff | 10/4/37 | 8/31/52 | 15 |
| Ernest M. Gruenberg | In Charge, Mental Health Program | 1/1/55 | 8/30/61 | 7 |
| Robin F. Badgley | Senior Member, Technical Staff | 5/1/63 | 6/30/68 | 5 |
| Per G. Stensland | Senior Associate | 7/1/67 | 9/1/73 | 6 |

### Past Semi- and Junior Professionals

| Name | Title | | | |
|---|---|---|---|---|
| Enid M. Shultes | In Charge, Publications | 11/25/25 | 4/20/61 | 36 |
| Katharine E. **Berry** | Member, Technical Staff | 2/27/28 | 5/31/65 | 37 |
| Xarifa (Sallume) Beam | Antioch Trainee | (1929) | (1932) | (3) |
| George A. Baker | Research Fellow | 10/1/29 | 5/29/30 | 1 |
| Elliott H. Pennell | Research Fellow | (1929) | (1931) | 2 |
| Victor O. Freeburg | Editorial Associate | 2/3/30 | 4/29/36 | 6 |
| Ruth L. Lewis | Technical Assistant | 12/16/30 | 12/31/37 | 7 |

## Past Semi- and Junior Professionals

| Name | Title at Retirement | Dates of Service | | Years of Service (Nearest Year) |
| --- | --- | --- | --- | --- |
| | | From | To | |
| Harry E. Seifert | Research Fellow | 5/26/32 | (1936) | (4) |
| Sally Preas | Technical Assistant | 3/15/37 | 12/31/46 | 10 |
| Robert B. Reed | Technical Assistant Research Fellow | 9/12/38 (1946) | 9/30/39 (1947) | 2 |
| Gilbert W. Beebe | Member, Technical Staff | 6/1/39 | 10/7/42 | 3 |
| Myron Kantorovitz | Research Associate | 1/23/40 | 12/31/42 | 3 |
| Anne Baronovsky | Technical Assistant | 2/9/42 | 9/26/47 | 5 |
| Louis Rubal | Technical Assistant | 7/13/42 | 12/10/62 | 20 |
| Marguerite Keller | Technical Assistant | 9/16/45 | 9/15/57 | 12 |
| Emily (Ketcham) Stamm | Nutrition Interviewer | 9/1/30 2/1/39 | 5/1/33 3/31/41 | 5 |
| Doris Tucher | Technical Assistant | 9/10/46 | 12/31/52 | 6 |
| Katherine Simon | Technical Assistant | 8/18/47 | 3/15/54 | 7 |
| Jane (Coulter) Mertz | Technical Assistant | 9/16/47 | 2/15/54 | 6 |
| Nathalie L. Schacter | Technical Assistant | 9/16/48 | 5/31/50 | 2 |
| Elizabeth (Jackson) Coulter | Research Associate | 12/13/48 | 8/15/51 | 3 |

| | | | | |
|---|---|---|---|---|
| Jeanne (Clare) Ridley | Technical Assistant | 4/8/49 | 9/30/52 | 3 |
| Charles F. Westoff | Research Associate | 9/29/52 | 8/31/55 | 3 |
| Erwin S. Solomon | Technical Assistant | 6/16/54 | 3/31/56 | 2 |
| Adelheid Wieland | Technical Assistant | 9/7/54 | 6/30/58 | 4 |
| Matthew Huxley | Administrative Assistant | 3/14/57 | 2/28/63 | 6 |
| Myrna E. Frank | Member, Technical Staff | 8/16/62 | 5/19/67 | 5 |
| Katherine C. Gensamer | Production Associate | 10/9/63 | 6/30/73 | 10 |
| Marguerite Schulte | Member, Technical Staff | 10/26/64 | 8/11/67 | 3 |
| Larry E. Blaser | Managing Editor | 10/14/65 | 4/30/73 | 8 |
| Ronald Szczypkowski | Research Associate | 12/1/68 | 9/15/71 | 3 |

### Present Professional and Technical Staff

| | | | | |
|---|---|---|---|---|
| L. E. Burney | Executive Director and President | 9/1/70 | Present | 4 |
| John S. Baugh | Executive Vice President, Secretary and Treasurer | 7/15/68 | Present | 6 |
| David P. Willis | Vice President for Program Development and Evaluation | 9/1/70 | Present | 4 |
| Richard V. Kasius | Associate | 4/1/53 | Present | 21 |
| Juan A. Inclan | Administrative Supervisor | 4/15/63 | Present | 11 |
| Florence Kavaler | Study Director (Chapel Hill Office) | 10/12/72 | Present | 2 |

# Name Index

Unless otherwise specified, Index relates to chapter numbers.